Essentials of Abdominal Ultrasound

Edited by Samia Ali Abdo Gamie and Enas Mahmoud Foda

Published in London, United Kingdom

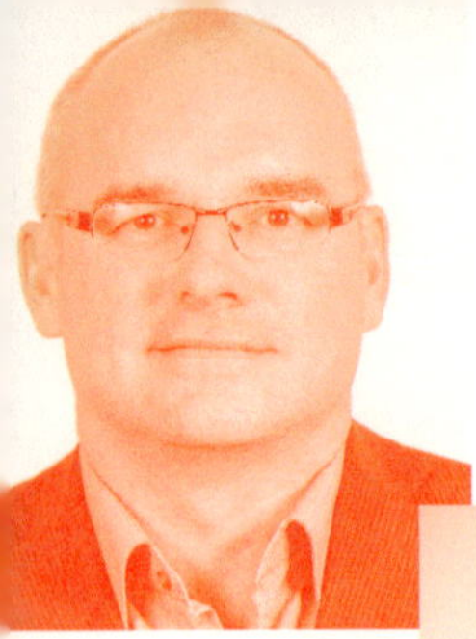
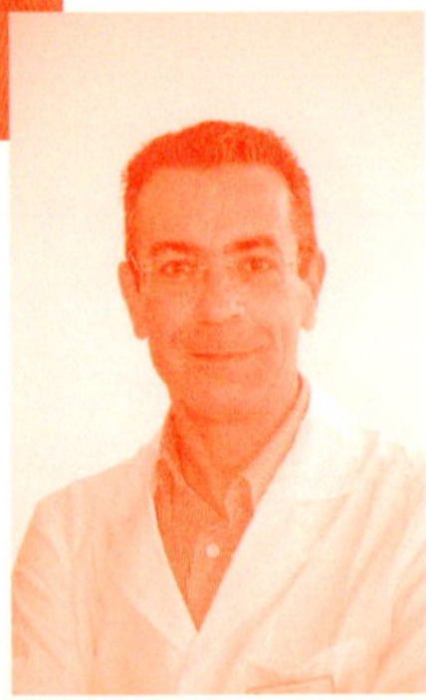
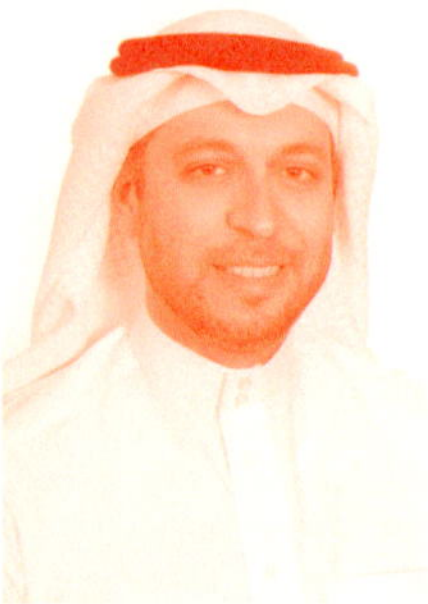
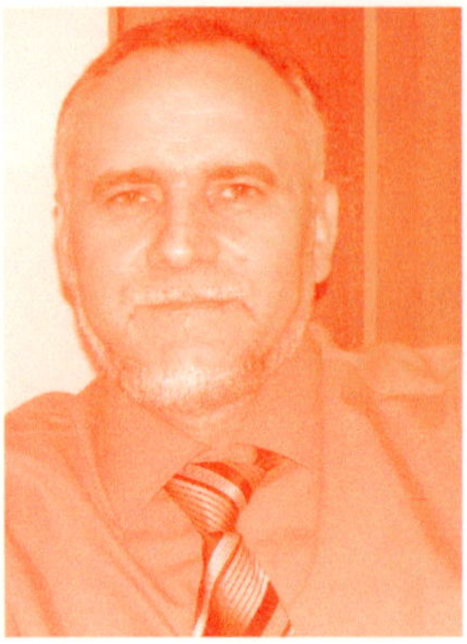
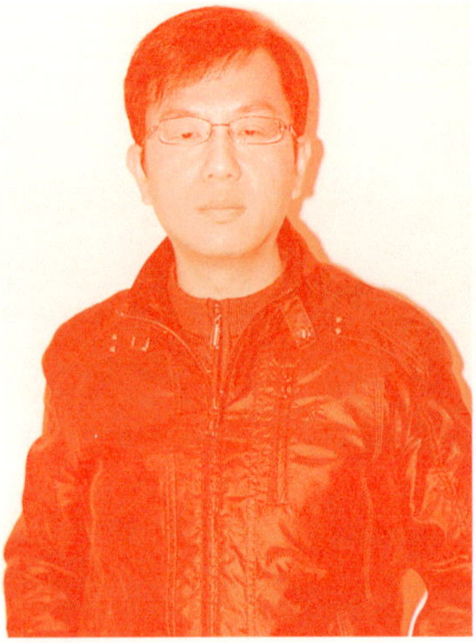
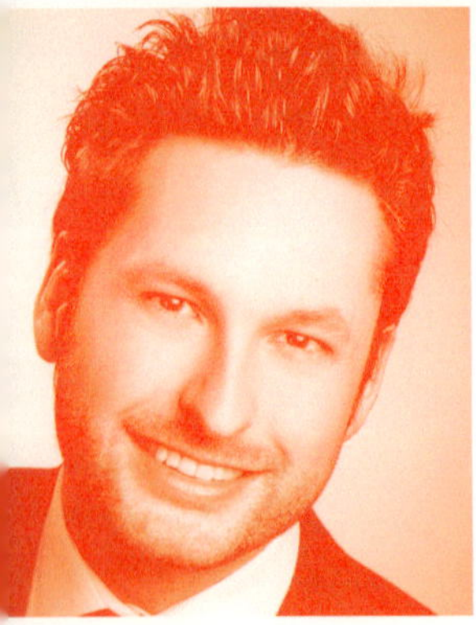
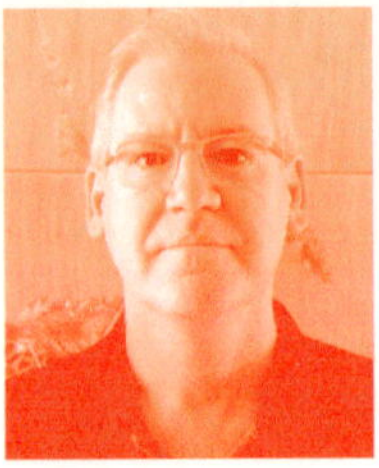

IntechOpen

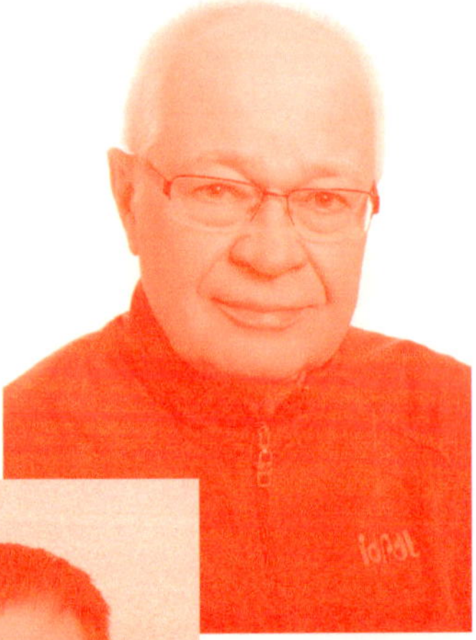
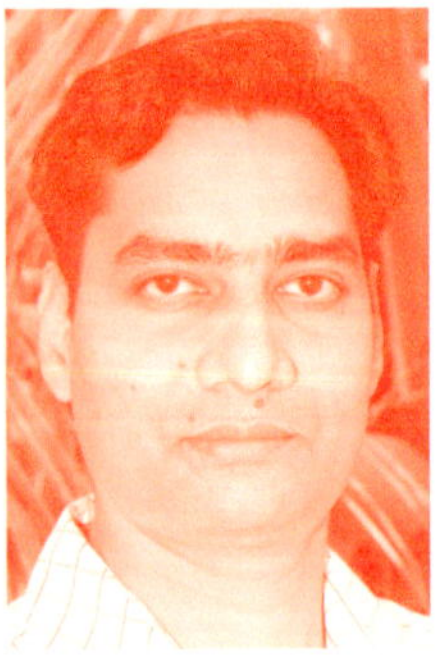
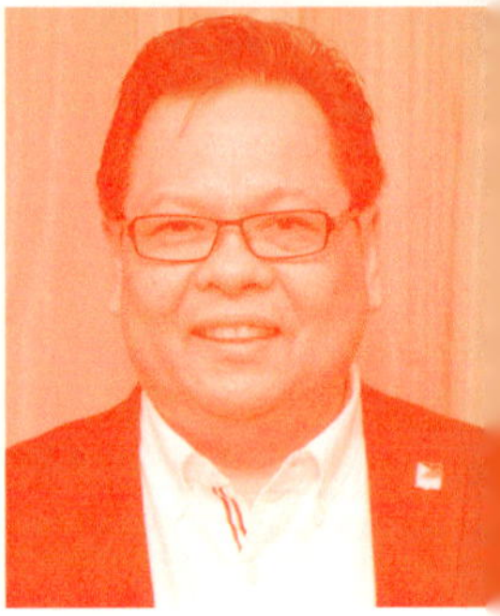
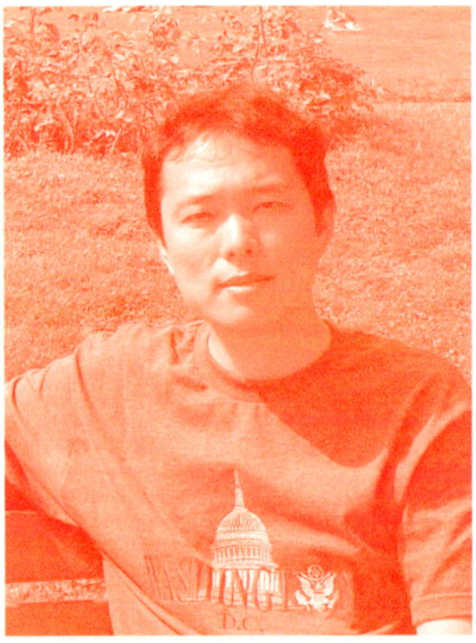
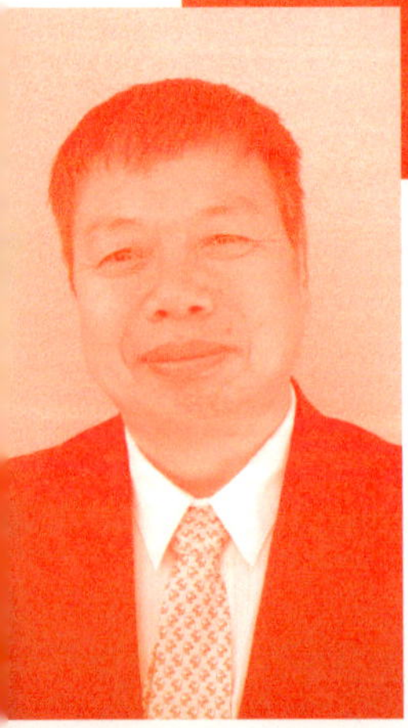
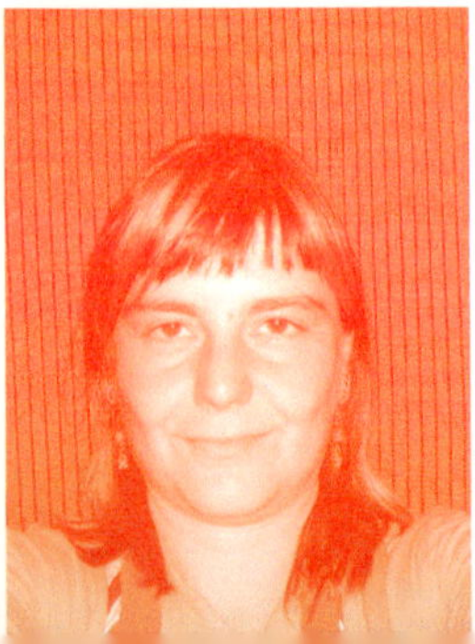

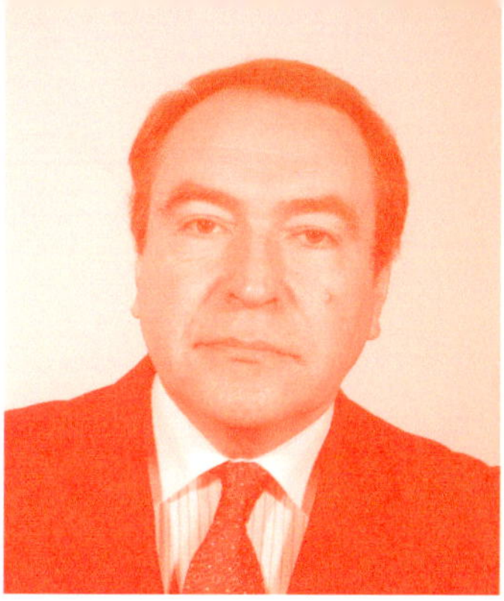
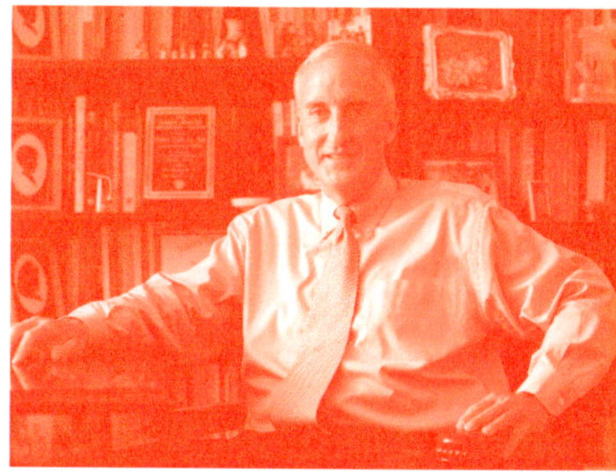
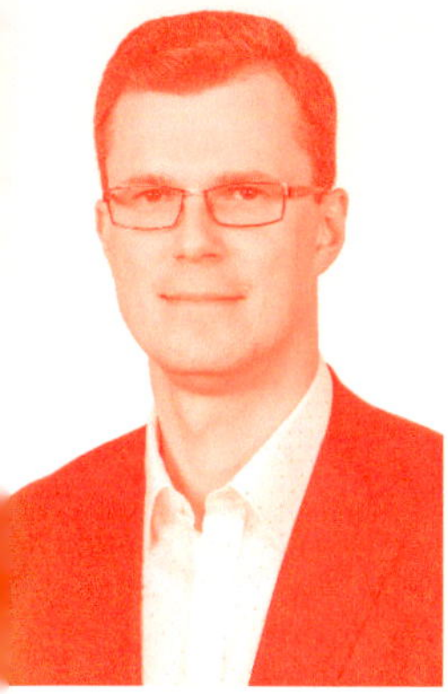
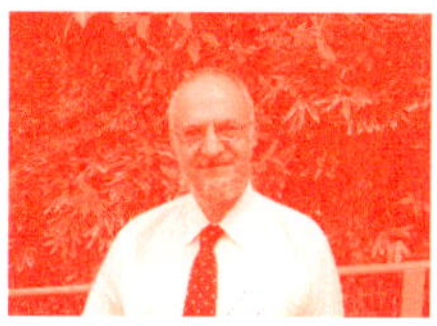
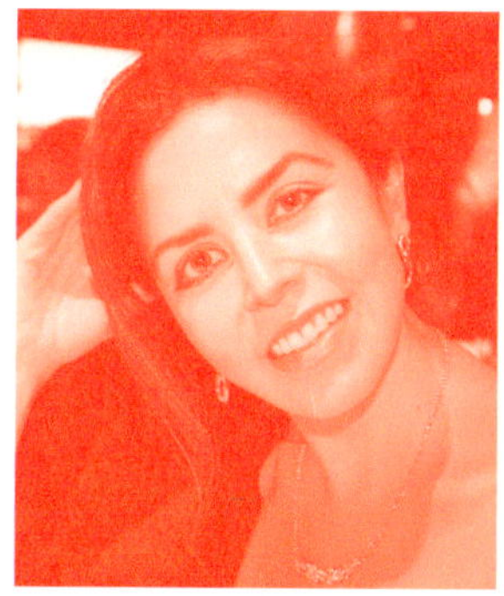

Supporting open minds since 2005

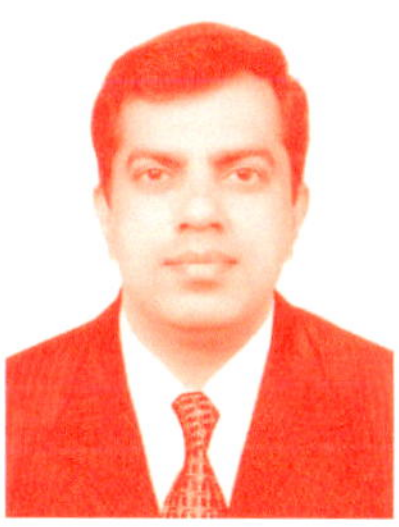
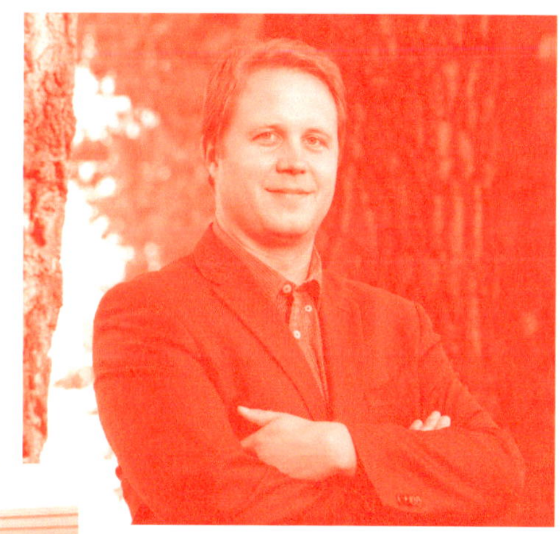
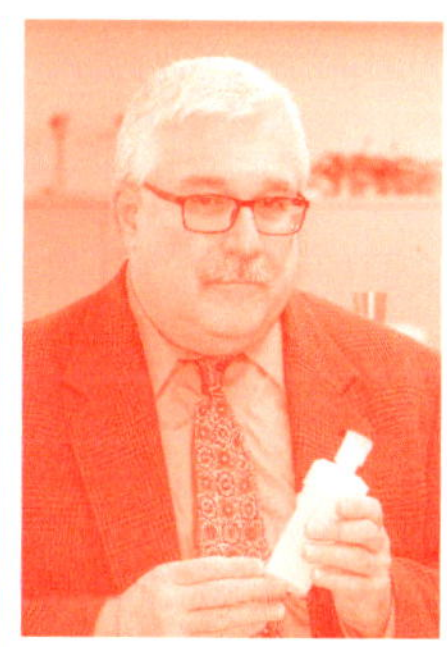
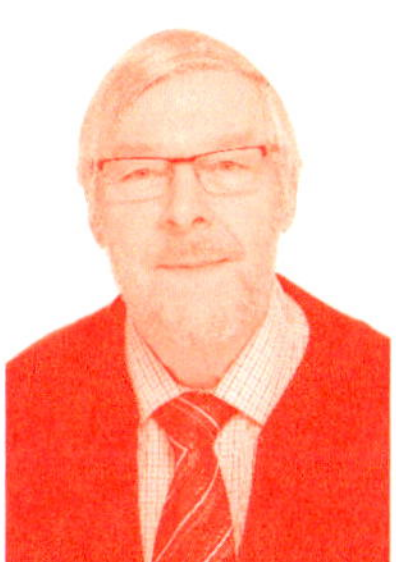
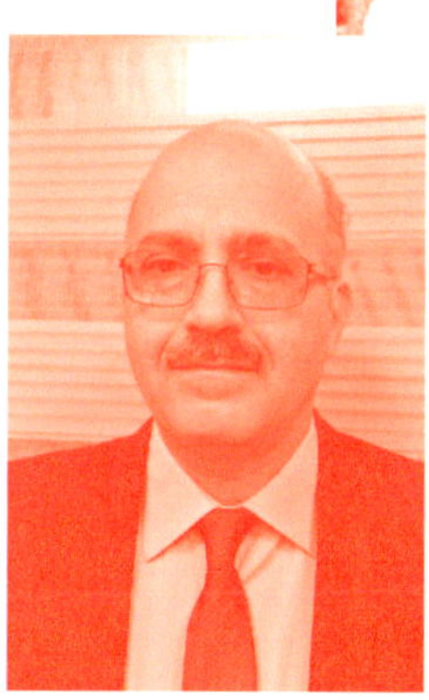
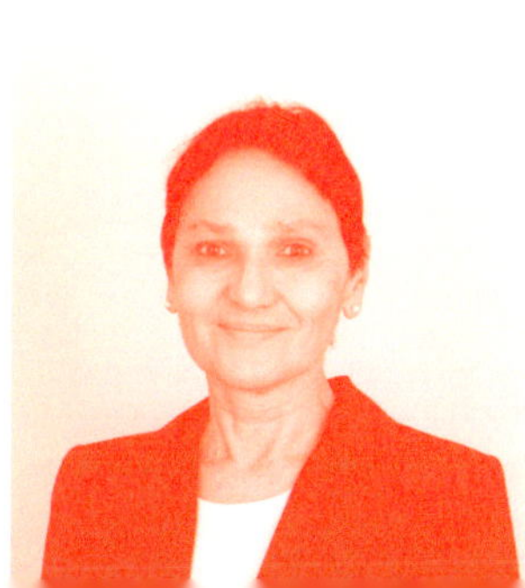
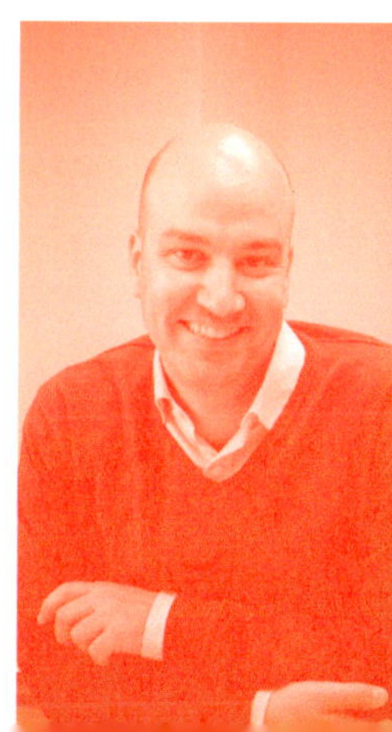

Essentials of Abdominal Ultrasound
http://dx.doi.org/10.5772/intechopen.73848
Edited by Samia Ali Abdo Gamie and Enas Mahmoud Foda

Contributors
Yaw Amo Wiafe, Augustina Badu-Peprah, Philip Njemanze, Daniel Fuster, Xavier Garcia-Calvo, Paola Zuluaga, Inmaculada Rivas, Arantza Sanvisens, Jordi Tor, Robert Muga, Moawia Gameraddin, Ercan Ayaz, Samia Ali Abdo Gamie

First published in London, United Kingdom, 2019 by IntechOpen
IntechOpen is the global imprint of INTECHOPEN LIMITED, registered in England and Wales, registration number: 11086078, The Shard, 25th floor, 32 London Bridge Street
London, SE19SG - United Kingdom
Printed in Croatia

British Library Cataloguing-in-Publication Data
A catalogue record for this book is available from the British Library

Additional hard and PDF copies can be obtained from orders@intechopen.com

Essentials of Abdominal Ultrasound
Edited by Samia Ali Abdo Gamie and Enas Mahmoud Foda
p. cm.
Print ISBN 978-1-78984-211-1
Online ISBN 978-1-78984-212-8
eBook (PDF) ISBN 978-1-78984-744-4

For EU product safety concerns:
IN TECH d.o.o., Prolaz Marije Krucifikse Kozulić 3, 51000 Rijeka, Croatia, info@intechopen.com or visit our website at intechopen.com.

Meet the editors

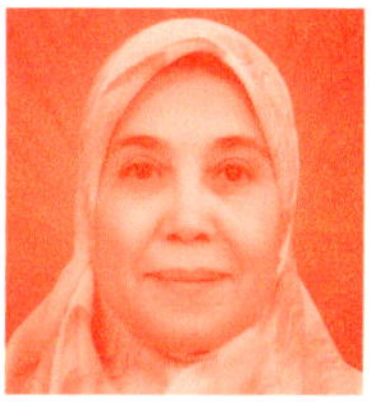

Samia Ali Abdo Gamie obtained her master's degree and PhD from Cairo Medical College. She is a professor of Internal Medicine at Helwan University, Egypt. She has trained individuals in the use of ultrasound for more than 20 years and organized the ultrasound training course for Ain Shams University Hospital, Egypt. She is a peer reviewer, author, member of the Egyptian Board Committee, and an examiner for the Egyptian Fellowship of Internal Medicine. Dr. Gamie is a member of the Medical Ethical Committee of Helwan University as well as director of the university's Student Assessment Service.

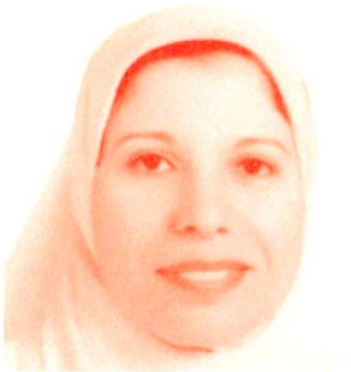

Dr. Enas Mahmoud Foda obtained her MD in Internal Medicine from Ain Shams University, Cairo, Egypt. She is professor of Internal Medicine, Gastroenterology and Hepatology at the same university. She also works in its Abdominal Ultrasound unit. Dr. Foda has presented at numerous conferences and is author of several published papers.

Contents

Preface

Abdominal ultrasound is a noninvasive bedside diagnostic tool that helps to discover many abdominal problems. It is safe and painless even in the early stages of pregnancy.

The development of ultrasound had its beginning in 1790 with the recognition of echolocation used by bats. Biologist Lazzaro Spallanzani first discovered that bats hear by listening for the return of the high-frequency sound they emit to detect objects and food. A breakthrough came in 1880 when physicist Pierre Curie and his brother Jacques Curie studied the properties of crystalline structure to demonstrate a piezoelectric effect, which was the scientific basis of the first transducer. This device generated a high-frequency sound and received its echo back. Ultrasound maps the body's structures based on the travel time and intensity of the ultrasound waves returning to the transducer from a given direction.

Diagnostic ultrasound began to be used in medicine for the first time during and shortly after World War II; the term SONAR (Sound Navigation and Ranging) was first used then as well. At that time, medicine began to realize the benefits of using ultrasound for detecting organ pathology.

The principle of ultrasound is to send ultrasound waves of particular frequencies into the body. When these waves meet the various structures of the body, the tissue will reflect, refract, absorb or transmit the wave. A special acoustic character can identify different tissue based on how much the tissue reflects or transmits the sound wave. Highly reflective structures show up as a white acoustic echo on the screen, while non-reflective structures appear as a black echo on the screen.

As we know, few people read a textbook from cover to cover. Most read one or more chapters that they find interesting. With this in mind, we designed the book so that each chapter provides complete, illustrative knowledge in itself. Each chapter is related to the scanning of one particular organ in the abdomen, and each organ is discussed from a different point of view. In each chapter, there is a new update of knowledge or technique. All chapters contain ultrasound images of real patients in recent work, and they are organized in the way that sonographers usually follow in scanning.

The content contained within this volume is relevant across many specialties, including radiology and internal medicine, and is useful for physicians and medical residents and students alike.

We want to express our deep thanks to the authors and mentors who gave their own time, effort and experience to write their chapters; they are clear, straightforward and organized. Mostly, we thank all of our patients who allowed us to use their information and be our main tool in this illustrative book. We hope that all our efforts will contribute to relieving your suffering and improving your health.

Last but not least, I would like to thank my beautiful, supportive family who has been by my side through every step. They truly are a blessing.

Samia Ali Abdo Gamie
Professor,
Pro of Internal Medicine,
Helwan University,
Cairo, Egypt

Enas Mahmoud Foda
Professor,
Pro of Internal Medicine,
Ain Shams University,
Cairo, Egypt

Section 1

Introduction

Chapter 1

Introductory Chapter: Common Pitfalls and How to Overcome

Samia Ali Abdo Gamie

1. Introduction

Medical ultrasound is an imaging modality using high-frequency sound waves to recognize unique tissue characteristics. The normal human range of audible sound is from 20 Hz to 20 KHz; in contrast the frequency used in medical ultrasound is >20,000 Hz. The frequency range that is used for medical imaging is generally between 2 and 18 MHz [1].

Piezoelectric effect discovered by Pierre and Jacques Curie in 1880 is the basic principle of ultrasound transducer. They discovered that when pressure is applied to quartz or some certain crystals, it creates an electrical charge in that material. Curie's brothers soon discovered the inverse piezoelectric effect; when an electric field was enforced onto crystal leads, it led to a disorder in the crystal lead—now called the inverse piezoelectric effect [2].

Piezoelectric transducer generates the ultrasound beam as a pulse travels through the tissue; the echo signals return to the transducer after undergoing absorption, reflection, and refraction depending on the tissue structure, leading to a real grayscale image formation. The basic rules in image formation can be summarized as follows. First, ultrasound pulse travels in a straight line, so echo signals travel in a narrow beam, giving a real-time scanning. Second, as the velocity of the ultrasound is constant, the distance is directly proportional to how far the structure is from the transducer. Third, the echo strength is related to the tissue reaction with the ultrasound waves; the reflected waves give the echo brightness on the screen that is referred to as tissue echogenicity [3].

Physics of the ultrasound is essential for all physicians to understand and interpret ultrasound images. Frequency is the number of the sound waves per second. It usually remains constant maintaining the frequency of the original source, but the velocity of the ultrasound wave changes depending on the physical properties of the medium. These variations in velocity introduce artifacts into the image, mainly attributed to bone and fat. The frequency of transducer determines the resolution of the ultrasound image. The resolution of the ultrasound machine is its ability to detect and display two close structures as distinct. Higher-frequency transducers have higher resolution, but its ability to penetrate to deep structures is low; therefore it is used for superficial structures. On the other hand, low-frequency transducers can penetrate to deep structures with lesser resolution; therefore it is suitable for deeper structures. Using high transducers of high frequency to screen deep structures results in more attenuation to the image of the deep tissue [4]. Choosing the proper transducer for a proper image of different organs is based on this rule of thumb regarding the transducer's frequency. Therefore, always use a sector transducer from 3.5 to 5 MHz to screen deep abdominal structures but higher frequency for superficial structures [5].

IntechOpen

Practical image orientation is performed in two planes sagittal plane and transverse plane. Using the transducer in the sagittal plane, the left side of the image represents the cranial plane. Meanwhile putting the transducer in a transverse plane, the left side of the image represents the right side of the patient. Abdominal examination is usually started while the patient is lying comfortably in supine position, and then they must be examined on both sides. Systematic scanning is important; scanning of all organs and all areas is essential to complete your mental checklist in an ultrasound report.

Preparation for abdominal ultrasound generally requires fasting for 8 h, decreasing the gas in the intestine. Also, for the gall bladder and biliary tree exploration, fasting is essential for screening. Other conditions such as emergency ultrasound require no special preparations. In each chapter of this book, if any special preparation for screening the organ is required, it will be mentioned.

In practice, ultrasound artifacts are common; thus understanding these artifacts' physics is vital to help correct it to improve the images, leading to good interpretation for a correct diagnosis. The artifacts arise either from improper operator technique or from the physics of ultrasound transmission and traveling. Identification of the artifact from improper technique is the first step, so it can be avoided. The second step is to know how the physics' artifacts can be corrected, keeping in mind that some of these artifacts may be good clues for proper diagnosis of structures with special characteristics. In this book, in each chapter, we try to explain some of these artifacts and how to avoid them. Potential US artifact correction is important for image quality improvement, optimal interpretation, and diagnosis.

Artifacts can be classified into two: One, related to the beam and the resolution, and the other, related to the location and the attenuation. Here are some common examples of these artifacts, their clinical relevance, their physical mechanism, and how to make alteration.

Beam- and resolution-related artifacts

Beamwidth artifact: Lateral resolution is the ability to detect two close points in the transverse plane as two distinct points. It leads to lateral blurring of the image and aberrant echoes from adjacent highly echogenic objects. It can be reduced by focusing the sound selection. Focusing improves the beamwidth, so it becomes narrower at the target focal zone [6].

Section thickness artifact: It is the ability to distinguish two vertical beams as two distinct points. It is called elevation resolution as the point planes are perpendicular to the transducer plane. It appears like debris in anechoic structure as cyst or ascites. It can be overcome by putting it in a focal zone with a standoff pad [7].

Secondary lobe artifacts: It mimics debris in anechoic structures. It is from the reflected echo that comes back from ultrasound waves that are transmitted outside the beam. It can be corrected by reducing the gain [8].

Location characteristics ultrasound artifact

Reverberation artifact: It appears as multiple bright parallel lines at regular intervals that decrease in intensity as the depth increase. It is due to reflections between highly reflective interfaces in parallel (reverberates). It may be useful in the detection of air in abnormal locations, as in pneumatosis, pneumoperitoneum, and pneumobilia. It can be reduced by decreasing gain, changing the angle of insonation, or using multiple windows [9].

Comet tail artifact: Adenomyomatosis, based on the same principle of reverberation artifact. It is caused by highly reflective interfaces that are closely spaced, so the individual echoes cannot be distinguishable. This artifact is useful as it considered a fingerprint for identification and diagnosis of cholesterol crystals in adenomyomatosis of the gallbladder (**Figure 1**) [10].

Ring-down artifacts: It arises from resonant vibrations within trapped air bubbles. These vibrations produce a continuous sound wave transmitted back to the transducer; it appears as a streak or series of parallel bands deep to a focus of gas. It can be useful in identifying abnormal foci of air, e.g., pneumoperitoneum and portal venous gas. Also, it can be indicative of appendicitis if it is detected in the appendix [11].

Mirror image artifact: It mimics disease, such as pseudo-thickened bowel wall and lesions in the lung. It is due to reflections of a highly reflective structure, e.g., the diaphragm, producing a mirror-like image of an object. The second image is generated along that path, deeper than the true site of the structure due to increased time of the return echo. A common example is in the case of a liver lesion near the diaphragm; the transmitted beam is reflected off the diaphragm and will be faced with a liver lesion that reflects it to the diaphragm again as well as the transducer. The image on the screen contains two lesions similar on both sides of the diaphragm and the same distance from it (**Figure 2**). This type of artifact may be corrected by decreasing gain or changing the angle of insonation [11].

Accentuation and attenuation characteristics of ultrasound artifacts

Increased transmission (accentuation): It is due to increased intensity of echoes distal to a low-attenuating structure. It is useful in practice to differentiate between cystic and solid structures. Distal to cystic structure there is an increased echo intensity, as the ultrasound waves pass through the cystic structure without any disturbance or loss. This accentuation is important to confirm the diagnosis of the anechoic cystic lesion (**Figure 3**). It can be increased by using tissue harmonic imaging [12].

Attenuation artifacts: Attenuation is a loss of ultrasound energy and amplitude as it goes deeper through the tissue. Therefore, echo from deeper structure comes weaker than the echo from the superficial structure; the ultrasound machine is computerized to amplify the return echo from the deeper structures. If the tissue is reflective, as in the case of a fat tissue, less echo reaches the deeper structure, and screening will be difficult. This attenuation is adequately compensated by first-order correction schemes such as time gain compensation.

Acoustic shadowing: It is due to a reduction in echo strength distal to a highly reflective object. Three types of acoustic shadowing, clean, partial, and dirty,

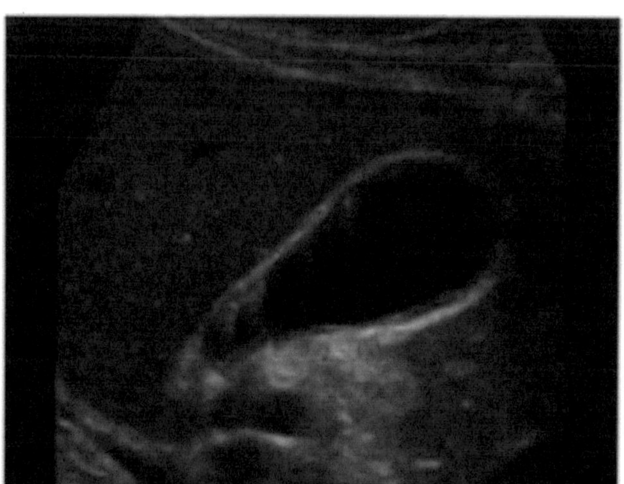

Figure 1.
Longitudinal US image of the gallbladder shows comet tail artifact caused by cholesterol crystals in Rokitansky-Aschoff sinuses. This finding is diagnostic of adenomyomatosis.

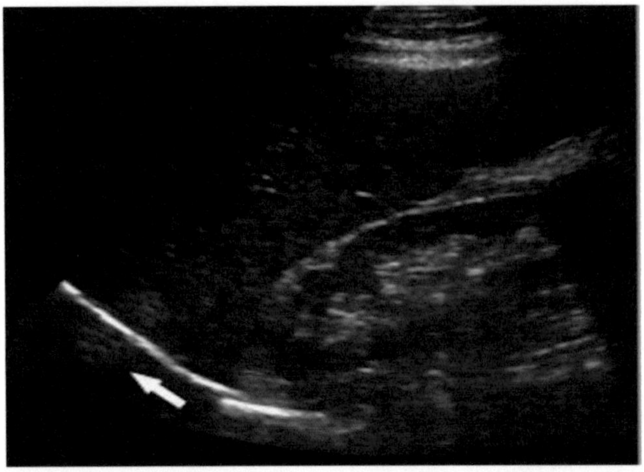

Figure 2.
Longitudinal US image shows an echogenic lesion in the right hepatic lobe (hepatic hemangioma), and a duplicated echogenic lesion (arrow) on the other side equidistant from the diaphragm mimics lesion in lung parenchyma.

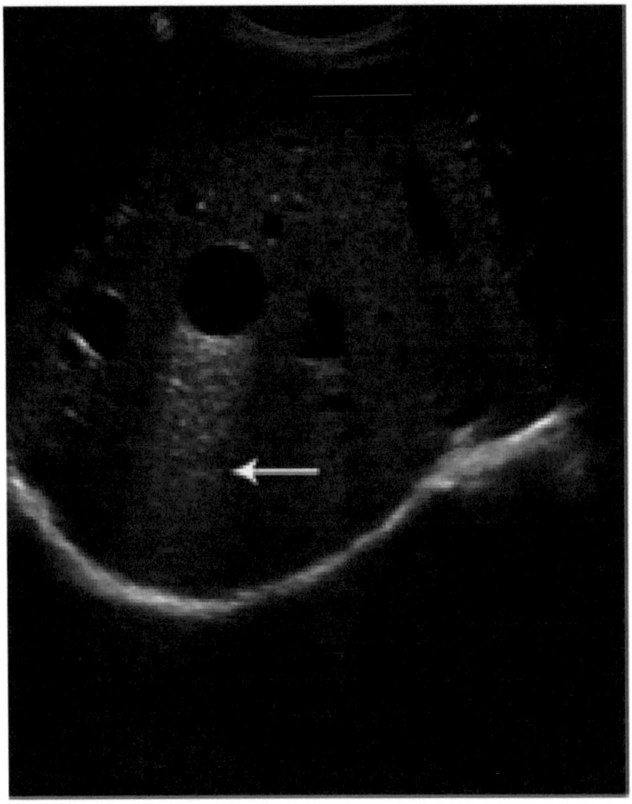

Figure 3.
Transverse US image of the liver shows anechoic hepatic cysts. The hepatic parenchyma distal to the cysts is falsely displayed as increased intensity (arrow) secondary to increased through-transmission artifact.

are used to describe the shadow of stones, calcification, and air, respectively. It is very helpful in practice to identify the clear shadow as a dark band due to all the ultrasound waves being absorbed. Its presence can help detect stones in echogenic structures such as kidney stones. Also, a shadow is important to differentiate a gall bladder (GB) stone (**Figure 4**), with its clear shadow, from a non-shadowing polyp or a sludge ball in GB. Dirty shadowing is seen in the case of highly refracting structure like gas. In clinical practice, it is important to increase the shadowing to help with the diagnosis of important pathology, so the focal zone and beam width are important to be adjusted in these cases [11].

The edge (refraction) artifact: It occurs in rounded structures like a cyst or urinary bladder as the ultrasound refracted at its edges results in shadows at both edges (**Figure 5**). These artifact shadows are corrected, and the shadows disappear by changing the angle of the ultrasound beam after identification of the artifact.

Anisotropy: It commonly occurs in tendons and, to a lesser extent, muscles, ligaments, and nerves. It appears as a hypoechoic area in a structure that has anisotropy. This phenomenon can be misinterpreted as a discontinuation of the course's structure. As the ultrasound beam is perpendicular to the tendon throughout its course, the tendon is uniformly hyperechoic. If the tendon is curved, the ultrasound beam is not perpendicular to the tendon; the tendon becomes hypoechoic and disappears. These phenomena can be overcome by changing the transducer position (heel-to-toe movement to make the transducer perpendicular on the tendon along its course) [13].

Understanding of these artifacts will minimize any misinterpretation in the report, and in certain situations it helps in the diagnosis. In this book, we used some of these artifact expressions for diagnosis or for explaining how to avoid any mistakes during scanning.

Standardized evaluation of abdominal ultrasound should optimally take place after overnight fasting in most of the ultrasound techniques; however, this is not a condition in urgent situations. In an emergency ultrasound, no special preparation is required. In routine clinical practice, fasting is important to avoid interfering bowel gas; also, it is recommended to assess the abdomen from a more lateral aspect through both flanks. Keeping in mind the need to take precautions, and being systematic in scanning, will provide clues to reach the correct diagnosis and avoid misinterpretation.

Starting ultrasound examination of the abdomen, it is usually done in a systematic manner. Your guide for scanning must be based on your mental checklist in the examination. Start by the right side considering the liver the acoustic window of the right upper quadrant of the abdomen. Go through the anatomical four areas of the abdomen, namely, the right upper quadrant, the left upper quadrant, the right lower quadrant, and the left lower quadrant. Intestinal loops can be screened in the

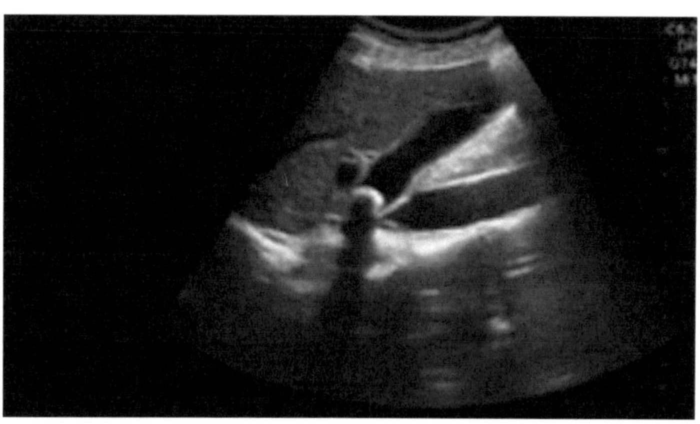

Figure 4.
Longitudinal US image of the gallbladder shows echogenic gallstones with clear shadow.

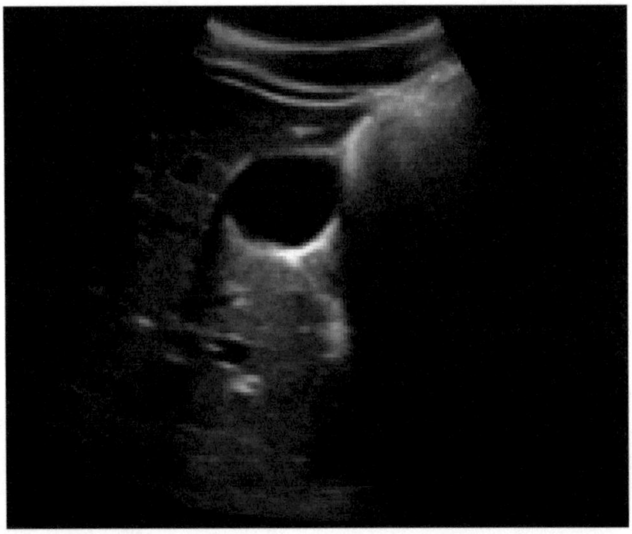

Figure 5.
Transverse US image of the liver shows transverse image of gallbladder with false shadow edge artifact.

"grid"-type pattern starting from the right side passing through the areas to the left side in a slow screening movement allowing to explore any intestinal pathology.

Ultrasound reports must fulfill all abdominal organs, with a full description of each in a systemic manner. A general outline of the sonographic description includes the architectures, the echogenicity of the parenchyma, and blood vessel distribution with a special comment on its variation from normal. The full screen of the organ is usually done with a complete orientation about the organ pathology. Any pathology is described as diffuse or localized, followed by detail descriptions of its site, size, echogenicity, regularity, and any special artifacts as mentioned above.

At the end of the report, there is a summary of the findings with your brainstorm conclusion. Ultrasound report is your mind checklist representing your systematic work and screening for the complete abdominal examination. Keep in mind that ultrasound findings are not histological but rather pathological. If from your clinical knowledge any additional investigation is required to confirm the diagnosis, it must be mentioned as a recommendation. Also, according to the ultrasound findings, a simple interventional process as ultrasound-guided biopsy procedures may be required. Also, good technical skills are needed for better interpretation of any valuable knowledge in the screening while avoiding the pitfalls and artifacts that can result in more confusion to the sonographers. In this text, many valuable technical skills are available from experts each in his field.

Author details

Samia Ali Abdo Gamie
Helwan University, Cairo, Egypt

*Address all correspondence to: samia_ali5@hotmail.com

References

[1] Hangiandreou NJ. AAPM/RSNA physics tutorial for residents. Topics in US: B-mode US: Basic concepts and new technology. RadioGraphics. 2003;**23**:1019-1033

[2] Genovese M. Journal of Diagnostic Medical Sonography Ultrasound Transducers. 2016;**32**(1):48-53

[3] Manbachi A, Cobbold RSC. Development and application of piezoelectric materials for ultrasound generation and detection. Ultrasound. 2011;**19**(4):187-196

[4] Abu-Zidan FM, Hefny AF, Corr P. Clinical ultrasound physics. Journal of Emergencies, Trauma, and Shock. 2011;**4**(4):501-503

[5] Szabo TL, Lewin PA. Ultrasound transducer selection in clinical imaging practice. Journal of Ultrasound in Medicine. 2013;**32**:573-582

[6] Bertrand PB, Levine RA, Isselbacher EM, Vandervoort PM. Fact or artifact in two-dimensional echocardiography: Avoiding misdiagnosis and missed diagnosis. Journal of the American Society of Echocardiography. 2016;**29**(5):381-391

[7] Hoskins PR, Martin K, Thrush A. Diagnostic Ultrasound: Physics and Equipment. 2nd ed. Cambridge: Cambridge, England; 2010

[8] Middleton WD, Siegel MJ, Dahiya N. Ultrasound artifacts. In: Siegel MJ, editor. Pediatric Sonography. 4th ed. Philadelphia, PA: Lippincott Williams & Wilkins; 2011. pp. 21-42

[9] Baad M, Lu ZF, Reiser I, Paushter D. Clinical significance of US artifacts. RadioGraphics. 2017;**37**:1408-1423

[10] Bonatti M, Vezzali N, Lombardo F, Ferro F, Zamboni G, Tauber M, et al. Gallbladder adenomyomatosis: Imaging findings, tricks and pitfalls. Insights into Imaging. 2017;**8**(2):243-253

[11] Feldman MK, Katyal S, Blackwood MS. US artifacts. RadioGraphics. 2009;**29**:1179-1189

[12] Rose JS, Bair AE. Fundamentals of ultrasound. In: Cosby KS, Kendall JL, editors. Practical Guide to Emergency Ultrasound. PA: Lippincott Williams and Wilkins; 2006. pp. 27-41

[13] Serafin-Król M, Maliborski A. Diagnostic errors in musculoskeletal ultrasound imaging and how to avoid them. Journal of Ultrasonography. 2017;**17**(70):188-196

Section 2

Knobology

Chapter 2

The Influence of Ultrasound Equipment Knobology in Abdominal Sonography

Yaw Amo Wiafe and Augustina Badu-Peprah

Abstract

Ultrasonography is a highly operator dependent imaging modality with a number of knobology variables that are under the control of the operator. Knobology is a terminology that describes the manipulation of ultrasound knobs and system controls in order to obtain the best image possible from diagnostic ultrasound. The inadequate use of knobology variables may impair image quality and can result in misdiagnosis. In abdominal sonography, selecting the appropriate application preset for abdominal examination is first step towards achieving an optimum image. The next step is to select an appropriate transducer frequency which must take the size of the patient into account. Transducer frequency is typically in the range of 3–5 MHz, but a lower frequency may achieve better depth penetration in larger patients. While the output power may improve image quality by increasing the intensity of transmitted sound energy, the impact is usually insignificant. The practice of using high output power should therefore be limited because of the risk of biologic effect. Other essential knobs for better image optimization include controlling the overall gain, time gain compensation, focal zone, dynamic range and tissue harmonic imaging. In the assessment of blood flow in abdominal vessels the regulation of the pulse repetition frequency, Doppler gain, imaging angle, and wall filter improves the sensitivity of color and spectral Doppler.

Keywords: knobology, resolution, greyscale imaging, Doppler imaging, ALARA principle

1. Introduction

Ultrasonography is a highly operator dependent imaging modality with a number of knobology variables that are under the control of the operator. Knobology is a terminology that describes the manipulation of ultrasound knobs and system controls in order to obtain the best image possible from diagnostic ultrasound. The inadequate use of knobology variables may impair image quality and can result in misdiagnosis.

This chapter explains the functions of the various ultrasound system controls and knobs and the impact they have on greyscale ultrasound imaging. It demonstrates the effect of transducer selection on image quality, and the role of knobology variables in image optimization. This includes a description of the Application Preset, Output Power, Overall Gain, Time Gain Compensation (TGC), Focus, Depth, Zoom, Dynamic Range and Tissue Harmonics. The influence of these essential knobs and system controls on spatial resolution (including lateral and axial resolution) and Contrast resolution are explained. In addition, the utility of Doppler knobs for imaging abdominal blood vessels are also explained and demonstrated.

The need to adhere to the principle of As Low As Reasonably Achievable (ALARA) is also explained with emphasis on the imaging of neonates and children. Lastly, the chapter also emphasizes the potential detrimental effect of underutilizing ultrasound knobs and system controls in abdominal sonography.

2. Switching-on the ultrasound machine

Switching on the ultrasound machine is the first knob to press if the machine is switched off. By switching on the machine, the ultrasound system is given access to a source of electricity, which excites the tiny piezoelectric crystals within the connected transducer. These piezoelectric crystals emit sound waves as a result of their exposure to electricity. The sound waves produced by the piezoelectric crystals can then be transmitted into the human body, normally aided by a coupling gel which serves as an acoustic medium for eliminating the air between the surface of the transducer and the skin.

3. Application preset

Modern machines allow the operator to preset an application setting for a certain examination type. Ultrasound imaging is used for a wide range of medical applications. Aside its use in assessing the abdomen, it is also used in obstetrics and gynecology, cardiac and vascular examinations, and other small-part examinations such as breast, thyroid, and musculoskeletal imaging. Different sonographic settings are needed for the various examinations, due to their differences in terms of the depth of region of interest, tissue-type, and the size of organs and structures in that region. Because of the uniqueness of these examinations, adjusting the settings between patients for a different examination can be time consuming, and may compromise the adherence to ALARA principles. In addressing this limitation, the manufacturer makes it easier by allowing the operator to select the type of examination which will activate the pre-defined factory settings for the specific type of examination. By selecting the appropriate 'Application Preset' for abdominal examination, the pre-defined factory settings are activated for abdominal sonography. This automatically adjusts the basic settings for the selected examination, which include an adjustment of the transducer frequency, acoustic Output Power, Overall Gain, Dynamic Range, Depth and other related settings.

Performing an abdominal ultrasound with a different application preset may impair the image quality which could mislead image interpretation. For example, a user performing an obstetric examination may identify a need for including abdominal examination without switching to the abdomen preset. This may impair the image quality of the abdominal examination if careful adjustments of relevant knobology variables are not made. In **Figure 1a**, obstetric preset was used in imaging the kidneys of an obstetric patient who complained of flank pain during an obstetric ultrasound examination. Upon using the basic obstetric preset without further manipulation of essential knobs, there was the tendency of suspecting a focal lesion in the right kidney (see arrow in **Figure 1a**). However, a switch to the basic abdomen preset without further manipulation resulted in an improved image quality which shows a normal kidney (see arrow of **Figure 1b** in the same person).

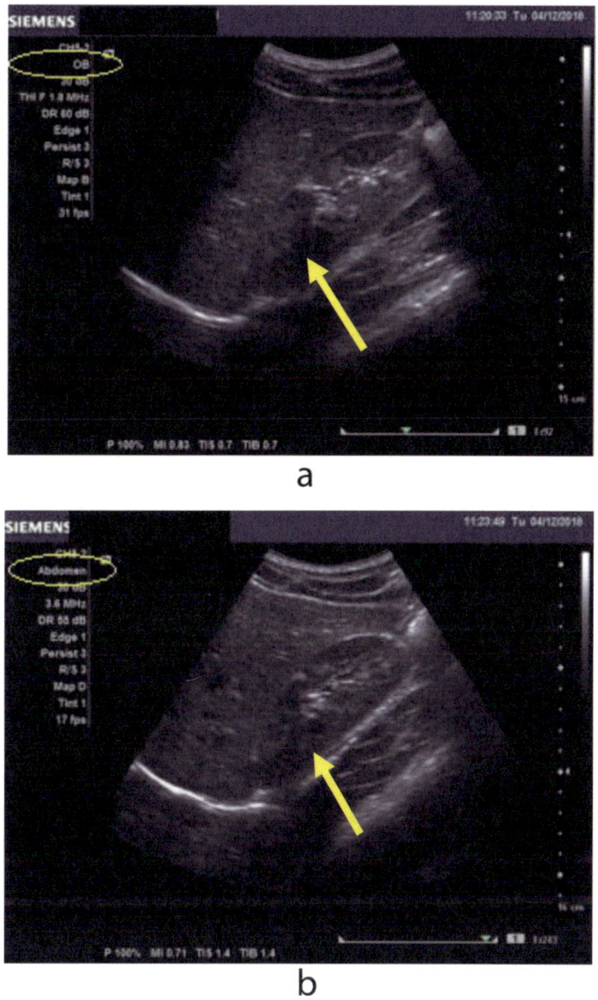

Figure 1.
(a) Image of the right kidney with OB preset suggests a focal change within kidney (see arrow). (b) Image of the right kidney with abdomen preset suggests normal appearance (see arrow).

It therefore suggests that much more manipulation of knobs will be required for selecting the 'wrong' application preset which may unduly extend the duration of the examination as a compromise on ALARA principles.

4. The transducer

Ultrasound images are produced from high frequency sound waves that are emitted by the transducer, typically in the range of 1–15 MHz [1, 2]. The frequency of the transducer is determined by the thickness of the piezoelectric crystals and the damping material behind them [3]. In producing a higher frequency, the manufacturer places a damping material behind very thin piezoelectric crystals in order to shorten the pulses of sound waves that are emitted [3]. However, shorter pulses of sound waves are unable to penetrate deeper because of shorter wavelength [3]. Due to this penetration limitation, different types of transducers are designed with different ranges of frequency. Higher frequency transducers offer better resolution at the expense of depth penetration, whilst lower frequency transducers offer better depth penetration for poorer image resolution [2, 3].

Since most abdominal organs such as the liver, spleen, kidneys, pancreas and aorta are relatively deeper, lower frequency transducers are used for this type of examination. Unlike the transducers designed for other examinations, the transducers for abdominal examination (i.e. sector or curvilinear) have a divergent and wider far field. Aside the lower frequency of curvilinear and sector transducers which makes image resolution relatively poorer, there is also an increase in attenuation as the sound beam travels deeper. This may adversely affect the image resolution of abdominal sonography. It is therefore incumbent on the operator to make a careful choice between better image resolution and depth penetration.

The typical frequency range for curvilinear transducers is in the range of 2-5 MHz. In selecting a frequency for an abdominal examination, the operator should consider the size of the patient. If the patient is smaller in size, a higher frequency should be used for better spatial resolution. Particularly in neonates and children, a higher frequency is highly useful, as this is likely to produce better image resolution to shorten the duration of the examination in fulfillment of ALARA principles. Secondly, children are less likely to cooperate during the examination, therefore using a lower frequency such as 3 MHz for abdominal examination may unduly delay the examination because of the lack of patient cooperation and a poorer image resolution. **Figure 2a** and **b** demonstrates two images of the right and left kidneys

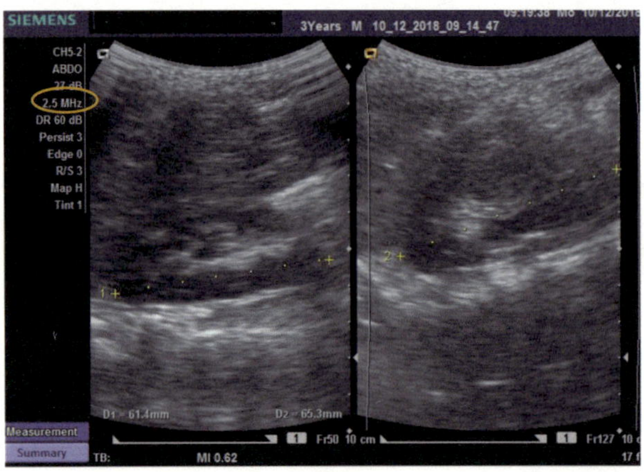

a

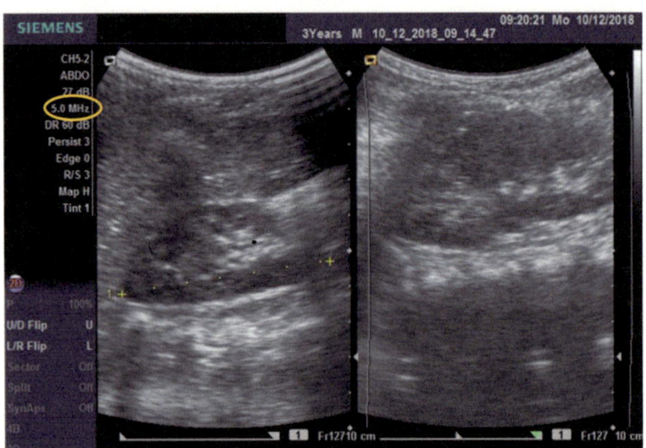

b

Figure 2.
(a) Image of the right kidney of right and left kidney in a 3-year-old non-cooperating patient showing poorer image resolution because of lower transducer frequency of 2.5 MHz. (b) Image of the right kidney of right and left kidney in the 3-year-old non-cooperating patient showing better visualization of renal margins because of lower transducer frequency of 2.5 MHz.

obtained from a 3-year-old infant with the higher frequency obviously showing more details than the lower frequency. However, a low frequency of 3-4 MHz is often ideal for imaging the average-sized adult, whilst larger or much more obese adults may require as low as 2 MHz of frequency for adequate depth penetration.

In addition, a linear transducer may also be used during abdominal ultrasound. Linear transducers use higher frequencies for imaging structures that are more superficial, such as the anterior abdominal wall and the surface of the liver. They are also used in assessing the appendix.

5. Output power

The acoustic output power of the machine must be considered at all times by the operator. As indicated above, selecting the appropriate preset for abdomen ultrasound will automatically adjust the output power to the recommended level. However, while it is important to observe the ALARA principle by using the minimum output power possible, the operator must not compromise image quality for output power reduction which may lead to misdiagnosis. In essence, there should be a balance between maximizing image quality with the minimum output power possible as a measure for reducing the risk of biological effect. Usually, the ultrasound

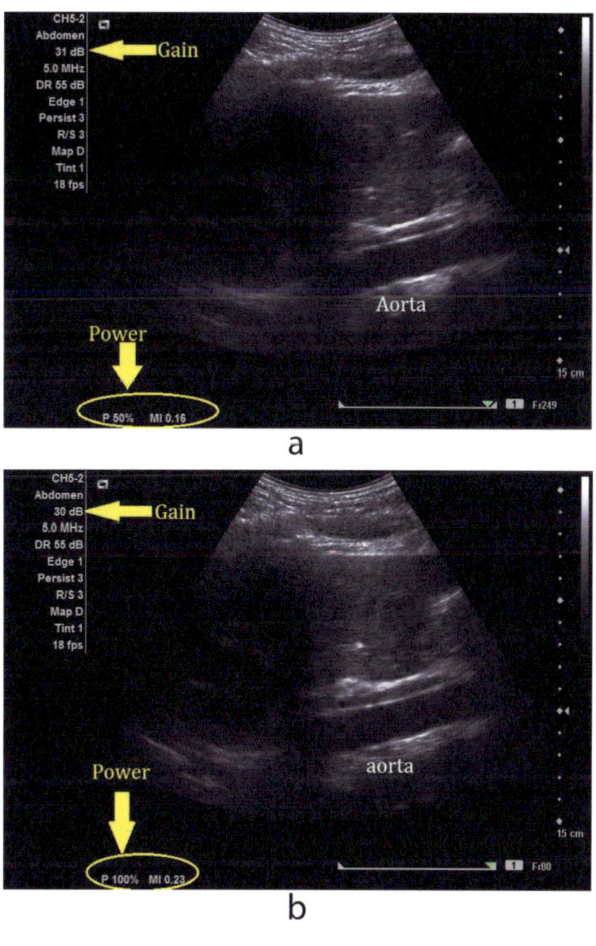

Figure 3.
(a) The appearance of the abdominal aorta at a reduced output power by 50%. (b) The appearance of the abdominal aorta when the output power increased was increased to 100 showed no significant difference %.

machine will display the output power on the screen at all times, allowing the operator to be constantly informed (**Figure 3a** and **b**). However, while increasing the power output may be useful, it may also be needless in many cases. The over-all Gain can play a better and safer role in image quality optimization than the output power. **Figure 3a** and **b** demonstrate that there is no significant difference between the appearance the abdominal aorta if the output power is reduced by 50% and the overall gain is about 30 decibels.

6. Overall gain

The overall gain is the recommended option to consider in place of increasing the output power. With the overall gain, image quality can be improved by adjusting the brightness of the entire field of view without increasing the intensity of transmitted sound energy. It achieves this by amplifying the echo-signals returning from the body after transmitting the sound waves. The overall gain can be considered as the 'microphone' in ultrasound imaging. The technology is similar to using a microphone to amplify someone's voice for the listener. Increasing or decreasing

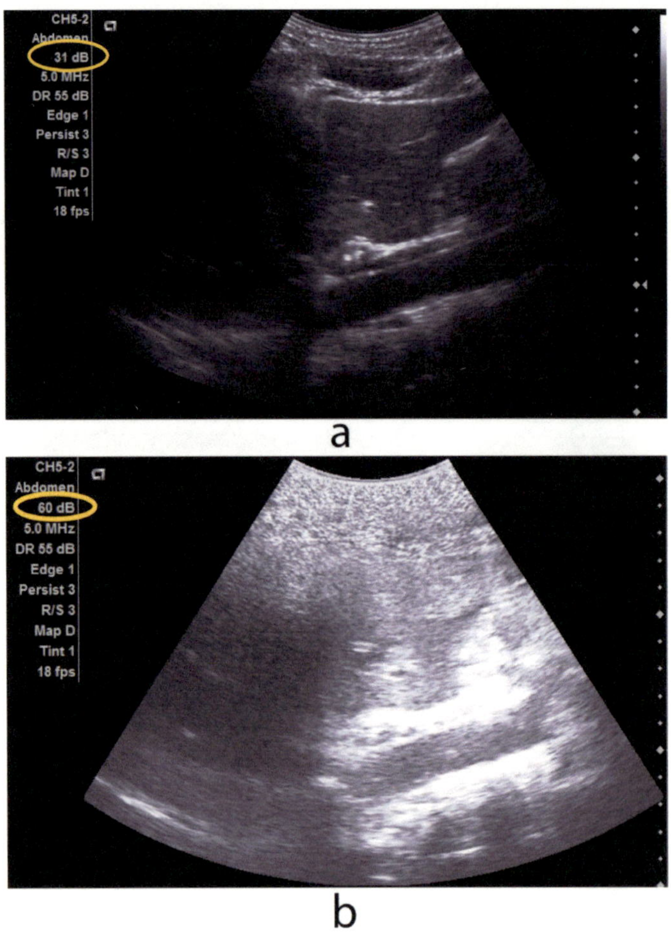

Figure 4.
(a) Adequate overall gain of 31 decibels with liver surface showing. (b) Too high overall gain of 60 decibels with liver surface missing.

the overall gain may improve contrast resolution for adequate visualization of the image. However, just as a microphone can sometimes produce noise and become a nuisance, increasing the overall gain beyond a certain point will affect contrast and spatial resolution by making the image appear too bright. Nonetheless, it is a knob you cannot do without in image optimization. Most modern machines integrate the overall gain in the Bmode or 2D knob, but it is still a separate knob in some machines. Manipulate the overall gain by adjusting it 'up and down' and carefully observe the changes that occur as you control the knob. **Figure 4a** and **b** shows images of adequate versus high overall gain and the effect it has on assessing the surface of the liver.

7. Time gain compensation

While the overall gain would adjust the brightness of the entire field of view, it may not address attenuation occurring at specific depths. Some structures in the body are much more affected by attenuation than others and would therefore need additional compensation for the loss of sound energy. For example, an optimum visualization of the left lobe of the liver requires a depth specific gain adjustment that is different from the gain compensation needed for optimum visualization of the right lobe. Hence the Time Gain Compensation (also known as Depth Gain Compensation), is a set of depth-specific slide controls that can be used for echo-signal amplification at different depths (see **Figure 5**). It allows the adjustment of echo-signals in the near-field, mid-field and far field to improve axial resolution. The TGC creates uniformity in the brightness of the echoes when used in conjunction with the overall gain. The best approach is to center all the TGC settings before adjusting the overall gain. After adjusting the overall gain, the TGC can then be adjusted to compensate for attenuation at specific depth.

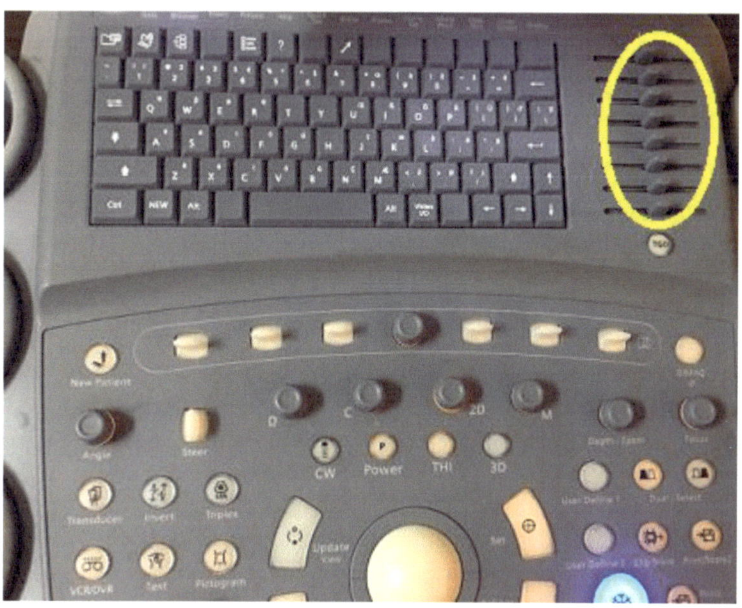

Figure 5.
TGC slide in the yellow circle.

8. Focal zone(s)

During scanning, the system allows the operator to improve lateral resolution in a region of interest by adjusting the focal zone. This is an additional measure to minimize the effect of attenuation. However, while other controls such as the overall gain and TGC are effective for improving axial resolution, adjusting the focal zone is much more effective for improving lateral resolution. Lateral resolution refers to the ability to identify structures lying side-by-side as separate structures, while axial resolution refers to the ability to identify a structure lying on another structure as separate structures.

The focal zone normally appears at the lateral side of Bmode as a triangular-shaped structure or a dot. It can be moved up or down by the operator and should be placed at the region of interest or posterior to that region. If a single focal zone is set too superficially a poorer image resolution will be observed in the far field (**Figure 6**). However if the focal zone placed below or at the level of region of interest, the resolution improves in the entire field of view (**Figure 6**). To improve lateral resolution in a wider region, more than one focal zones may be selected by the operator. However, increasing the number of focal zones also decreases the frame rate which has the tendency of slowing down the image production time to the detriment of temporal resolution. Thus using more focal zones slows down the scanning time which may not support the principles of ALARA in terms of keeping to a reasonable scanning time.

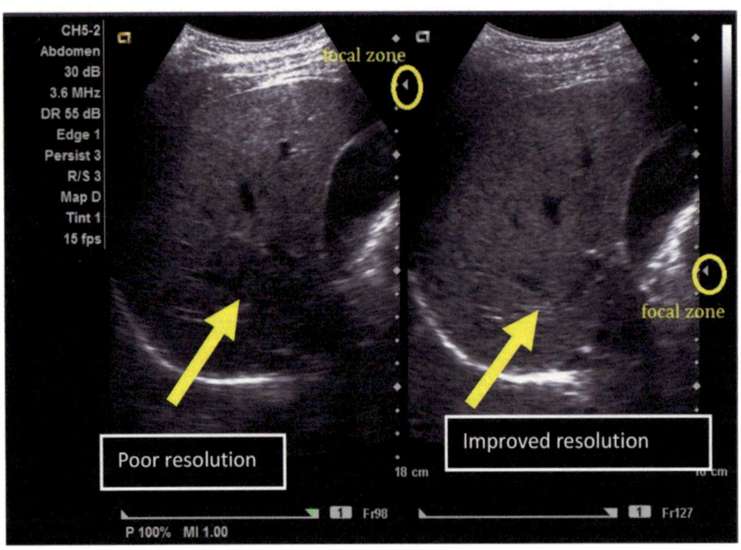

Figure 6.
Poorer resolution when focal zone is positioned in the near is compared to focal zone positioned at the level of interest.

9. Depth

The Depth is special a knob for adjusting the distance of the field of view. Structures within the field of view can be moved far or closer by adjusting the Depth. This is to ensure that the region of interest is closer enough for optimum visualization. It is also to avoid showing regions that are not relevant to the area of interest. **Figure 7a** is an example of a far depth image of the pancreas, with a wide irrelevant space showing behind the spine. This irrelevant space can be avoided by adjusting the

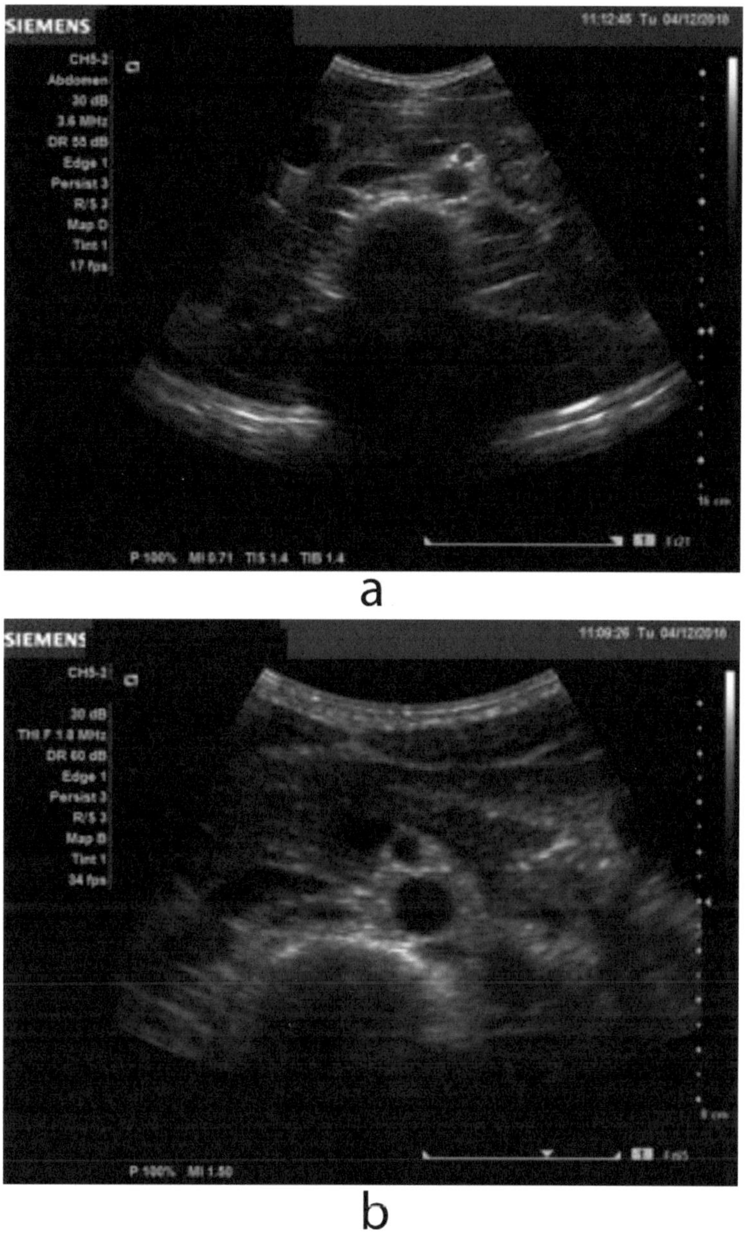

Figure 7.
(a) Far depth. (b) Closer depth.

Depth closer for adequate visualization (**Figure 7b**). The structure of interest should always take the center stage by occupying about two-thirds of the field view. In order to avoid missing a pathology beyond the field of view, the best practice is to adjust the Depth for a far field of view before adjusting for a closer field of view. **Figure 8** is an example of how one can miss a pathology, if the Depth is not adjusted for adequate visualization beyond the field view. It demonstrates how a closer Depth would have missed the pleural effusion if a far depth image was not assessed.

However, while moving the depth closer and far is necessary for evaluating various conditions and ruling out pathologies, moving the Depth closer has the tendency of generating noise which can worsen contrast resolution and may even mimic a pathology.

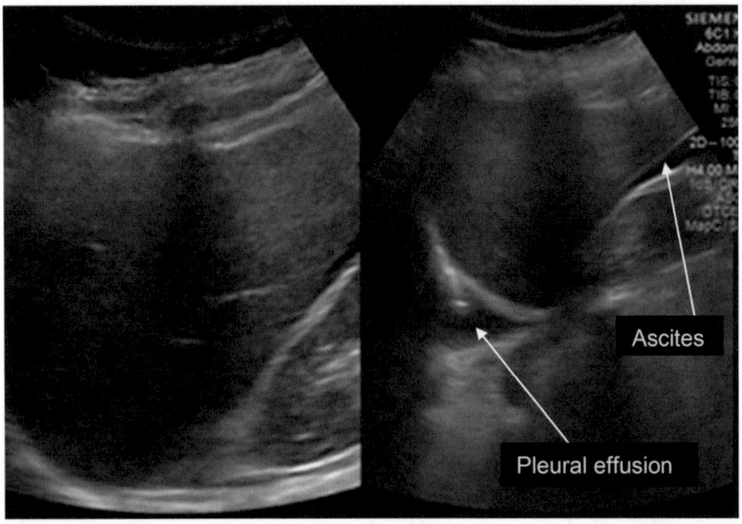

Figure 8.
Missing information on the right-side because of depth adjustment.

10. Zoom

The zoom is used for magnifying the area of interest. Unlike the depth which magnifies by moving the area of interest closer, the zoom actually magnifies by making the region of interest appear bigger. Another limitation of the depth that is

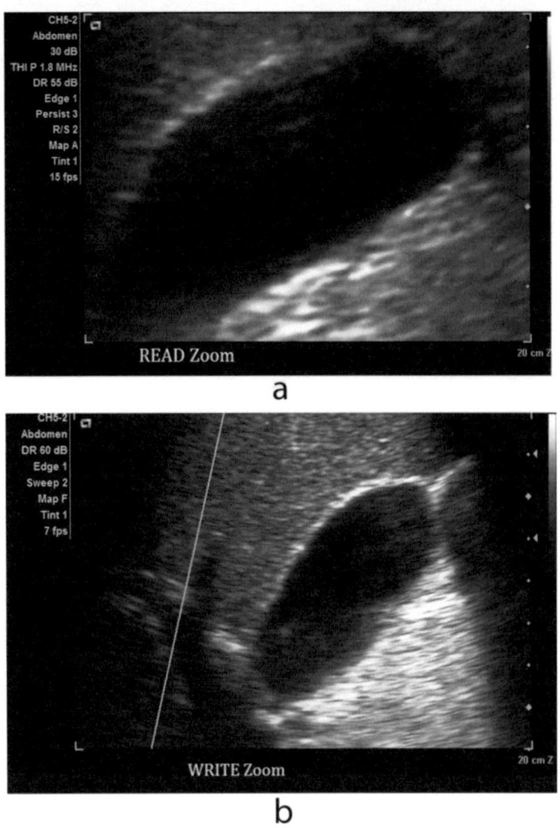

Figure 9.
(a) Read zoom. (b) Write zoom.

addressed by the zoom is the ability to enlarge a specific region of interest. Without using the zoom, measuring some tiny structures may difficult because of poor spatial resolution. For instance, in measuring the thickness of the gallbladder wall, using the zoom improves the visualization of the wall for an accurate measurement (**Figure 9a** and **b**).

Some manufacturers use READ zoom for their magnification, while others use WRITE zoom. Both read zoom and write zoom can produce poorer image depending on the size of the area magnified. However, READ zoom produces the worse kind of images because it relies on stored images which enlarges the pixel density in that region (**Figure 9a**). On the other hand, WRITE zoom tries to maintain the pixel density by zooming the image live which produces a better spatial resolution. Operators should check the type of zoom in their machine in order to appreciate how much zooming can be done without compromising the image quality.

11. Dynamic range

The Dynamic Range is a control on the ultrasound system that allows the operator to determine the range of shades of gray to be displayed on the monitor. Broad shades of gray displays a wider range of echo-intensity between bright and

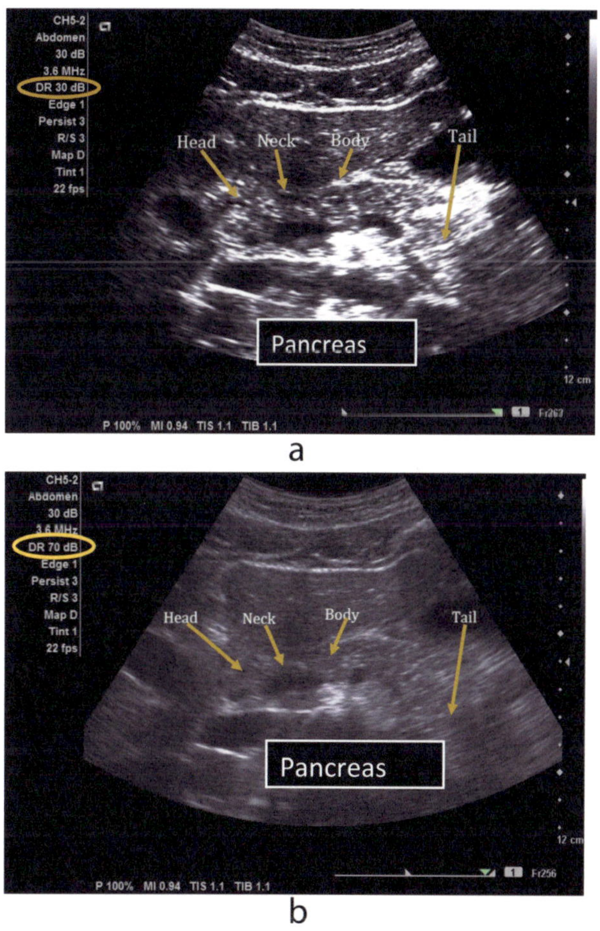

Figure 10.
(a) Narrow dynamic range. (b) Broad dynamic range.

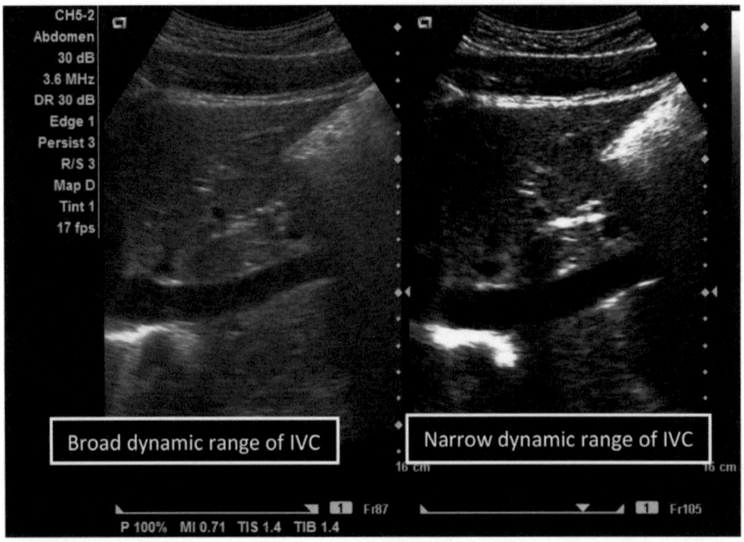

Figure 11.
Broad versus narrow dynamic range of IVC.

dark and produces a smoother image overall, whilst narrow shades of gray displays a narrower range of echo-intensity between bright and dark and produces a higher contrast between two regions of different echogenicity. In abdominal sonography, a broad dynamic range is the most appropriate option for assessing the echotexture of homogeneous soft-tissue structures like the liver, pancreas and spleen. Narrow dynamic range is most appropriate for assessing anechoic structures such as the aorta and IVC. **Figure 10a** shows the effect of narrow dynamic range of the pancreas in comparison to the liver, and **Figure 10b** shows the effect of broad dynamic range on the pancreas which shows poor differentiation in echotexture in comparison to the liver. In **Figure 11** also shows the effect of long and short dynamic range on the appearance of the IVC.

12. Tissue harmonic imaging

Tissue harmonic Imaging (THI) is an additional control for image optimization in most ultrasound machines. It improves image quality by eliminating weak echoes that cloud the image when the fundamental frequency of the transducer is used. It replaces the returning echoes from the fundamental frequency with echoes in the harmonic frequency which improves spatial resolution. This eliminates side lobe artifacts and noticeable noise in the area of interest. It can therefore be used in conjunction with the utilization of other knobs that may generate noise. For example, noise generated by increasing the Depth can be instantly eliminated by activating THI. **Figure 12** also shows an increase in noise as a result of increasing the overall gain and Depth, and how it is instantly eliminated by the activation of THI. The activation of the THI in **Figure 12** instantly changed the settings from the fundamental frequency to the harmonic frequency. In **Figure 13**, you also appreciate the importance of THI, in terms of how it improves visualization of the margins of liver surface in comparison with the adjacent image which did not use THI.

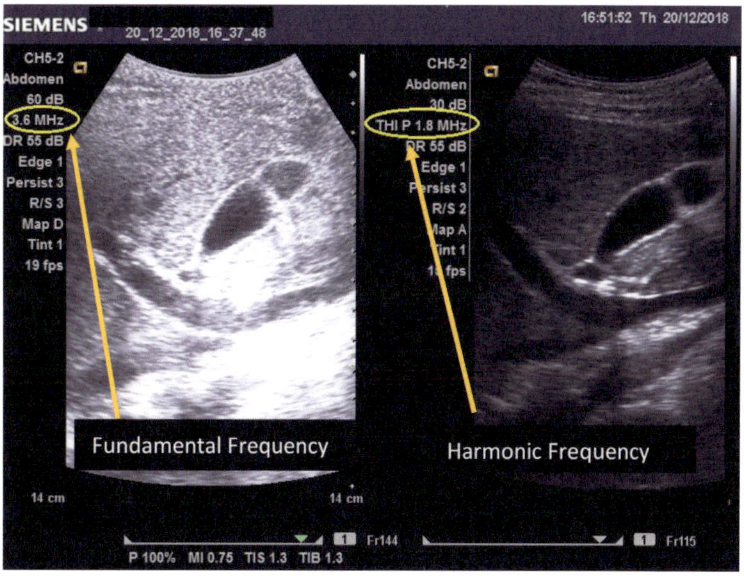

Figure 12.
Noise from increased overall gain and depth is instantly eliminated THI activation.

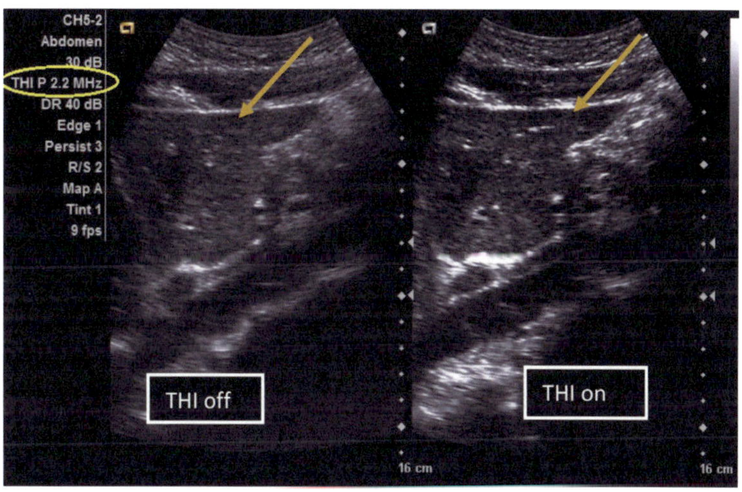

Figure 13.
Improved liver margins with activated THI.

13. Freezing and cineloop

The ultrasound machine also has a freeze button which enables the operator to stop and evaluate the image quality before storage. Saving an image without freezing implies that the image was not evaluated for quality. Freezing the image before storage is therefore recommended.

The cineloop is additional control that helps with selecting the best of the image frozen image. It displays image frames acquired in the last few seconds prior to freezing. The cineloop can be highly useful when scanning children.

14. Additional controls for imaging abdominal blood vessels

An abdominal ultrasound examination may also require the assessment of blood vessels and Doppler evaluation of blood flow. The fundamental knobs that influence both color and spectral Doppler imaging include the Doppler gain, pulse repetition period (PRF), and the wall filter. In assessing the presence of flow in smaller blood vessel, the minimum standard is to adjust the system for a higher Doppler gain, a lower PRF and a lower wall filter [4]. Careful manipulation is used in balancing these knobs, as a slight overlap between them can generate noise artifacts.

Figure 14a shows the poorer flow in the hepatic vein in comparison to the portal vein as a result of higher PRF. This is much improved in **Figure 14b** with decreased PRF.

In larger abdominal blood vessels such as the aorta, additional knob controls that are highly relevant include the imaging angle which must not be parallel to the surface of

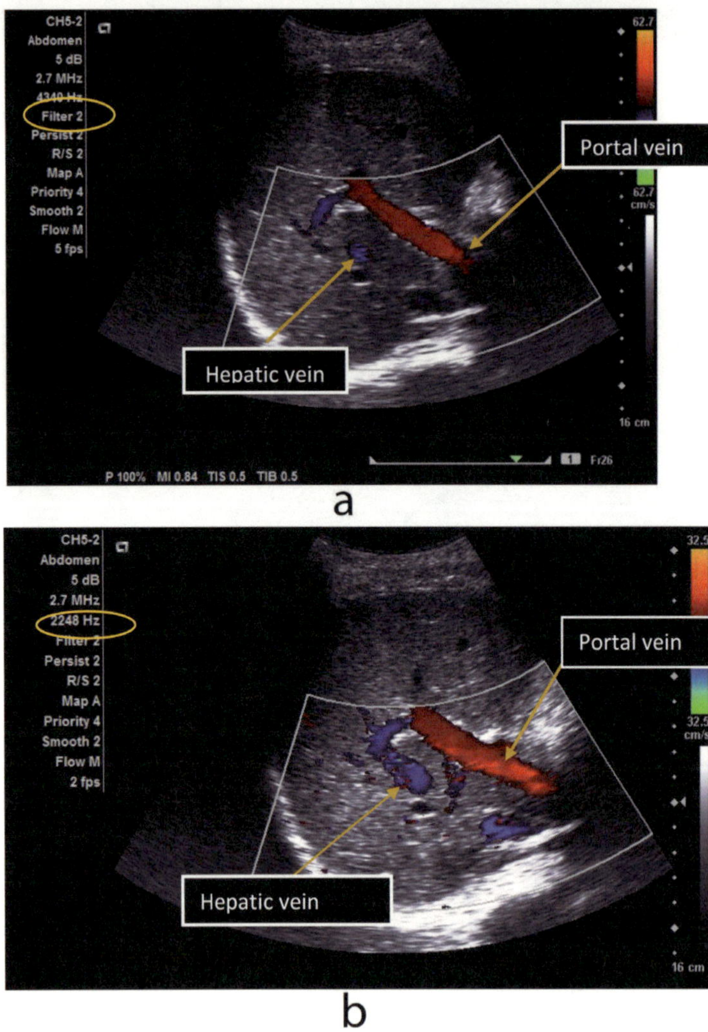

Figure 14.
(a) High PRF with low flow sensitivity in hepatic vein. (b) Low PRF with high flow sensitivity in hepatic vein.

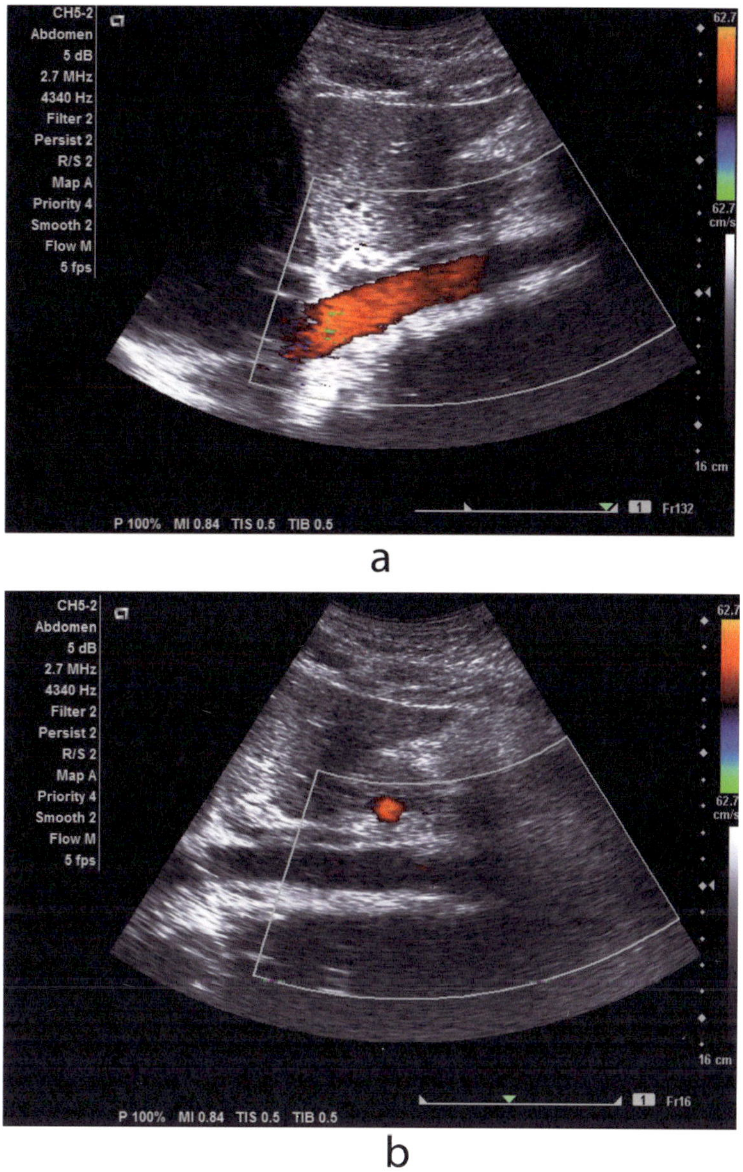

Figure 15.
(a) Color flow showing in angled vessel. (b) Color flow absent in parallel vessel.

the transducer. **Figure 15a** and **b** shows the effect of imaging angle on color flow in the aorta which is absent when the vessel is parallel to the surface of the transducer.

In spectral Doppler Imaging, however, lower PRF may cause aliasing artifact, especially when the baseline is high [5]. This can be corrected by increasing the PRF of the spectral waveform and lowering the baseline. **Figure 16a** shows aliasing artifact of the Superior Mesenteric Artery (SMA) which was as a result of a lower PRF and a higher baseline. By increasing the PRF and lowering the baseline, a normal waveform of the SMA was obtained in **Figure 16b**. Other essential knobology settings which improves spectral waveform in the assessment of peak systolic velocity include using a smaller sample gate and ensuring an angle correct setting that aligns with the vessel wall as demonstrated in **Figure 16a** and **b**.

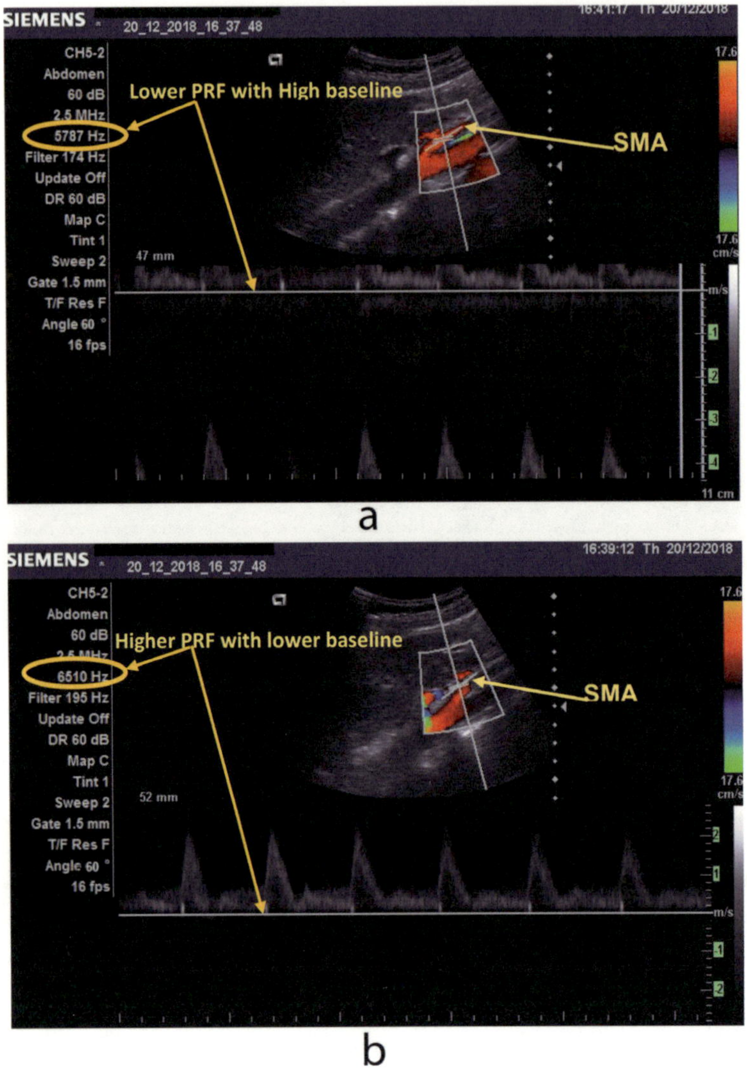

Figure 16.
(a) Aliasing artifact in the superior mesenteric artery as a result of lower PRF and higher baseline. (b) Adequate waveform for assessing peak systolic velocity in the superior mesenteric artery, after increasing the PRF and lowering the baseline.

15. Conclusion

Understanding the influence of knobology in ultrasound imaging is essential in abdominal sonography. The image quality can be optimized by selecting the appropriate application preset and transducer frequency. While using the highest output power may be useful, it is not necessary in many instances. The various knobology variables with direct influence on greyscale and color Doppler should be regularly manipulated by the operator for the best image possible in abdominal sonography.

Author details

Yaw Amo Wiafe[1*] and Augustina Badu-Peprah[2]

1 Medical Imaging Section, Department of Medical Diagnostics, Kwame Nkrumah University of Science and Technology, Kumasi, Ghana

2 Department of Radiology, Komfo Anokye Teaching Hospital, Kumasi, Ghana

*Address all correspondence to: wadart1@gmail.com

References

[1] Merritt C. In: Rumack CM, Wilson SR, Charboeau JW, Levine D, editors. Diagnostic Ultrasound. 4th ed. Mosby: Elsevier; 2011. p. 3. Ch. 1

[2] Venables H. How does ultrasound work? Ultrasound. 2011;**19**(1):44-49. DOI: 10.1258/ult.2010.010051

[3] Kremkau FW. Diagnostic Ultrasound: Principles and Instruments. Philadelphia, USA: WB Saunders Company; 2005

[4] Kim MJ, Kim KW, Kim SY, Kim JK, Won HJ, Shin YM, Kim PN, Lee MG. Technical essentials of hepatic doppler sonography. Current Problems in Diagnostic Radiology. 1 Mar 2009;**38**(2):53-60. Available from: https://doi.org/10.1067/j.cpradiol.2007.08.008

[5] Kruskal JB, Newman PA, Sammons LG, Kane RA. Optimizing doppler and color flow US: Application to hepatic sonography. Radiographics. May 2004;**24**(3):657-675. Available from: https://doi.org/10.1148/rg.243035139

Section 3

Liver Ultrasound

Chapter 3

Liver Ultrasound Abnormalities in Alcohol Use Disorder

Daniel Fuster, Xavier Garcia-Calvo, Paola Zuluaga, Inmaculada Rivas, Arantza Sanvisens, Jordi Tor and Robert Muga

Abstract

Alcohol-related liver disease is the most common alcohol-related medical illness, and it is the major driver of liver-related deaths worldwide. However, no screening guidelines currently exist for the early detection of liver disease in patients with risky drinking or those with alcohol use disorder. Moreover, most patients with alcohol-related liver fibrosis, which is the main prognostic factor of progression to end-stage liver disease, have normal blood tests. Abdominal ultrasound is a cheap and readily available diagnostic procedure that is rarely used in patients with alcohol use disorder without overt liver disease. In addition, abdominal ultrasound can detect other forms of liver disease, which are not uncommon in patients with unhealthy alcohol use, and can have a negative impact on the natural history of alcohol-related liver disease. In this chapter we will review the current knowledge about the use of liver ultrasound in patients with alcohol use disorder for the early detection of alcohol-related liver disease, as well as the potential use to detect other forms of liver disease. We will also briefly discuss other methods for the noninvasive detection of liver steatosis and/or liver fibrosis in patients with alcohol use disorder.

Keywords: abdominal ultrasound, alcohol-related liver disease, alcohol use disorder, liver steatosis; cirrhosis

1. Introduction

According to the last update of the Global Burden of Disease Study, alcohol consumption is the seventh leading risk factor for both death and the burden of disease and injury [1]. Besides tobacco, alcohol accounts for a higher burden of disease than any other drug, and alcohol-related liver disease is the most common alcohol-related chronic medical illness [2]. In recent years, there has been a worldwide increase in liver-related mortality due to end-stage liver disease [3], mostly because of the impact of alcohol consumption [4, 5]. With the recent advances in hepatitis B and C treatment, alcohol-related liver disease has become the main cause of liver-related mortality [6].

It is important to note that, compared with other forms of liver disease, alcohol-related liver disease has received little attention in the literature, as it is often stigmatized as a self-inflicted disease [7]. This is also true in clinical practice, as alcohol use is often not properly screened or accounted for in medical charts, both in primary care and hospital settings [8], and treatment for alcohol use is offered to a minority of patients [2].

In this chapter, after a brief introduction about generalities of alcohol-related liver disease and about the assessment of alcohol use in patients with liver disease, we will discuss the current evidence for the use of abdominal ultrasounds in patients with alcohol use disorder (AUD). The current evidence includes a recently published Cochrane review and our own experience with the systematic performance of abdominal ultrasounds in otherwise healthy adults with AUD admitted for hospital detoxification.

In addition, we will also discuss other potential benefits of the use of abdominal ultrasound to detect other forms of liver disease, which are not uncommon in patients with unhealthy alcohol use. We will address the use of liver ultrasound for hepatocellular carcinoma surveillance in patients with alcohol-related liver cirrhosis. Finally, we will include a brief mention of other available methods to screen for alcohol-related liver steatosis and alcohol-related liver fibrosis.

2. General overview of alcohol-related liver disease

Liver disease in patients with AUD encompasses a spectrum of histological abnormalities that includes steatosis, steatohepatitis, fibrosis, cirrhosis of the liver, and hepatocellular carcinoma [9, 10]. Those abnormalities, rather than being different stages of the disease, can coexist in the same patient. Acute alcoholic hepatitis is a severe complication that can occur at any point in the course of alcohol-related liver disease and is associated with liver failure and with high short-term mortality [2].

Alcohol-related liver steatosis in the absence of alcoholic hepatitis is potentially reversible with the cessation of alcohol consumption, but continued alcohol use is associated with progressive liver damage and an increased risk of alcoholic hepatitis [11]. Therefore, abstinence is advisable for patients with AUD and any form of alcohol-related liver disease, as it tends to diminish portal hypertension even in the more advanced forms of the disease [2]. Active alcohol consumption is a formal contraindication for liver transplantation, which is of concern as alcohol-related liver disease is the leading cause of liver transplantation in Europe [12].

A timely diagnosis of liver disease in apparently asymptomatic patients with AUD contributes to a better prognosis and facilitates treatment [13, 14]. In patients with unhealthy alcohol use, liver damage is a major driver of disease burden, and it is often diagnosed in advanced stages, including decompensated liver cirrhosis [14]. In fact, nearly 75% of patients with liver disease present for the first time with a nonelective hospital admission due to end-stage liver disease [5].

The use of liver ultrasound is recommended by the current European guidelines to promote an early detection of nonalcoholic steatohepatitis [15]. However, no guidelines exist for the screening and early detection of liver damage in unhealthy drinkers, and screening approaches in this population are currently a matter of debate [16, 17].

Therefore, there is a need for screening and early detection of alcohol-related liver disease in patients who drink alcohol in excess, as it is well established that sharing abnormal findings suggestive of liver disease with patients can trigger behavioral change and decrease the use of alcohol [18].

Moreover, surveillance aimed to detect hepatocellular carcinoma in patients with alcohol-related liver disease is suboptimal, and liver cancer is often diagnosed at a later stage when potential curative treatments are futile [10].

DOI: http://dx.doi.org/10.5772/intechopen.85941

3. Assessment of alcohol use in patients with suspected liver disease

The Alcohol Use Disorders Identification Test (AUDIT) is a validated tool for identifying AUD in patients [19]. AUD encompasses both alcohol dependence and alcohol abuse [20], and represents the more extreme form of unhealthy alcohol use [21]. The use of AUDIT is recommended by both the American Association for the Study of Liver Diseases (AASLD) and the European Association for the Study of the Liver (EASL) guidelines [22, 23]. Other options are AUDIT-C (a shorter version of the AUDIT) [24], and the single-question screening tool that has been validated for the screening in primary care of unhealthy alcohol use, that is, the spectrum of alcohol use that goes from risky alcohol use to AUD [25].

Patients who screen positive for unhealthy alcohol use merit further assessment to rule out health consequences of alcohol with an emphasis on alcohol-related liver disease [2]. Besides laboratory testing, we believe that the performance of an abdominal ultrasound can be useful in this setting [17].

In addition, referral of patients to physicians who are specialists in addiction medicine is an option to increase the chances of successfully remaining abstinent [2].

4. General overview of abdominal ultrasound for the study of liver diseases

Abdominal ultrasound is a cheap and widely available technique that is not usually performed to detect subjacent liver abnormalities in patients with AUD without overt liver disease.

4.1 Normal ultrasound findings of the liver

Abdominal ultrasound is an accurate method for estimating liver size, which should be determined at the midclavicular line and in normal conditions is less than 16 cm [26]. The liver parenchyma should be evaluated for focal and/or diffuse abnormalities. The normal liver appears as homogeneous with an echogenic texture. In normal conditions, liver echogenicity equals or slightly exceeds that of the renal cortex. This comparison heavily relies on the visual perception of the observer and on the presence (or absence) of disease processes in the renal cortex [27].

The right and left lobes, as well as the caudate lobe can be identified with the use of an ultrasound [28]. Other structures that should be identified are the main lobal fissure, which separates the left and right lobes and appears as an echogenic line that extends to the gallbladder fossa; the falciform ligament, which divides the left lobe into the medial and the lateral segments and appears as an echogenic area in the left lobe; and the ligamentum venosum, which separates the caudate from the left lobe and appears as an echogenic line anterior to the caudate lobe [28].

An abdominal ultrasound can also identify the major hepatic and perihepatic vessels, including the inferior vena cava (IVC), the hepatic veins, the main portal vein, and the right and left branches of the portal vein [28]. The main portal vein is characterized by thick and echogenic walls and enters the liver at the hilum. It divides into the right and left portal branches, and the left branch then divides into medial and lateral branches. The hepatic veins, which drain in the inferior vena cava, have thinner walls in comparison to the portal vein [28]. In addition, abdominal ultrasound is a reliable method for a first-line evaluation of portal vein abnormalities suggestive of portal hypertension [29]. It is also very useful to evaluate the biliary tree and to detect ascitic fluid, and it can also be used to guide the performance of a paracentesis [28].

Doppler evaluation should be used to document blood flow characteristics and blood flow direction, which is crucial in the diagnosis of portal hypertension [30]. In addition, Doppler evaluation can distinguish nodular lesions that are suggestive of hemangiomas, of hepatocellular carcinoma, or of liver metastases [31].

Figure 1 shows how a normal liver appears in an abdominal ultrasound.

4.2 Liver ultrasound in alcohol-related liver disease

In abdominal ultrasounds, liver steatosis appears as hyper-echogenicity due to the increased parenchymal reflectivity that intracellular fat accumulation produces [32]. The sensitivity of abdominal ultrasound to detect liver steatosis is impacted by the amount of fat content and severely decreases if fat content is lower than 10–20% [14].

The results about the ability of liver ultrasound to differentiate between liver steatosis and liver fibrosis have been mixed [33–35], and it is easier to differentiate when the degree of liver fibrosis is higher, as there is an increase in coarse echoes without posterior beam attenuation [32, 33, 36].

How to quantify liver steatosis with abdominal ultrasound is also a matter of debate. Liver steatosis is often classified as "mild," "moderate," or "severe" based on hyper-echogenicity, the discrepancy between echo amplitude in the liver and the kidney, impaired visualization of hepatic vessels, and loss of echoes from the walls of the portal system [36, 37].

Many authors consider steatosis to be *mild* if there is presence of hyper-echogenic liver tissue with fine and tightly packed echo targets and of normal beam penetration with normal visualization of the diaphragm and portal vein borders [38].

If there is decreased beam penetration with slightly decreased visualization of the diaphragm and the portal vein borders as well as moderate or diffuse increase of echo intensity, liver steatosis would then be considered to be *moderate* [38].

If there is a marked increase in echogenicity with no visualization of the portal vein border, an obscured diaphragm and posterior portion of the right lobe, and reduced visibility of the kidney, liver steatosis would be considered *severe* [38].

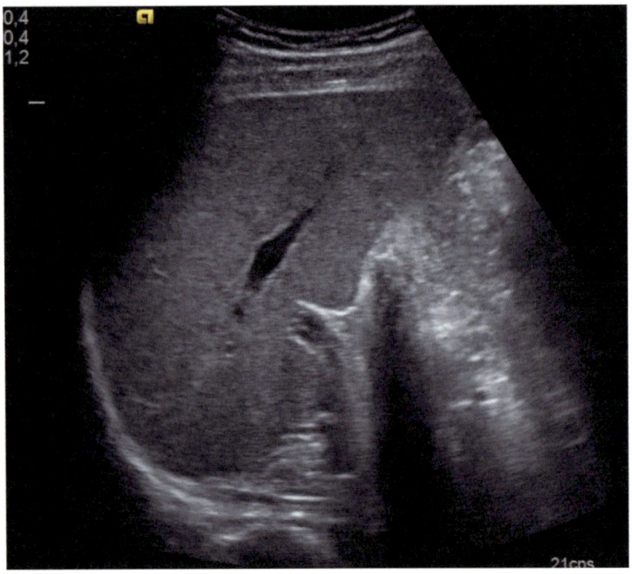

Figure 1.
Normal liver.

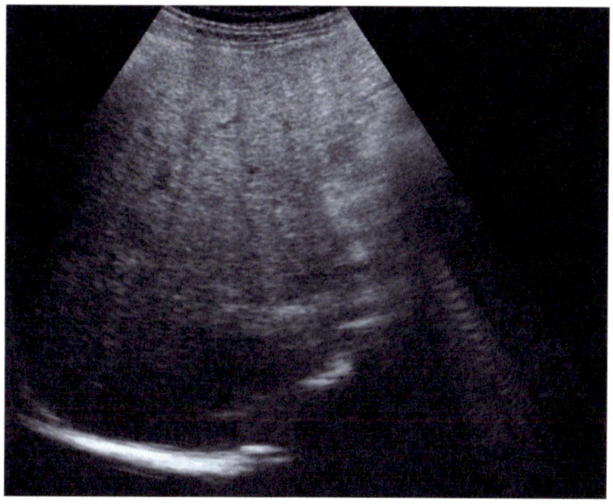

Figure 2.
Severe steatosis in an heterogeneous liver.

As mentioned in the introduction, different alcohol-related liver disease abnormalities can coexist in the same patient. **Figure 2** shows an abdominal ultrasound consistent with severe steatosis in a patient with AUD admitted for hospital treatment that also harbors a heterogeneous liver.

A potential weakness of liver ultrasound is operator dependency in assessing liver steatosis [27]. In a retrospective study that used static images of liver ultrasounds and included 168 patients from routine clinical practice and three independent radiologists, the mean inter-observer agreement rates for the presence of liver steatosis were 72%, while the mean intra-observer agreement 1 month later was 76% [27]. In that study, intra-observer agreement for the severity of liver steatosis ranged from 55 to 68% [27].

In general, there is agreement that abdominal ultrasound is a cheap and reliable method to identify moderate or severe liver steatosis [38], but its accuracy for mild forms of steatosis is lower and may increase with the use of a computer-aided method [38]. Besides liver steatosis, ultrasound findings that contribute to the detection of alcohol-related liver disease include (among others) liver size,

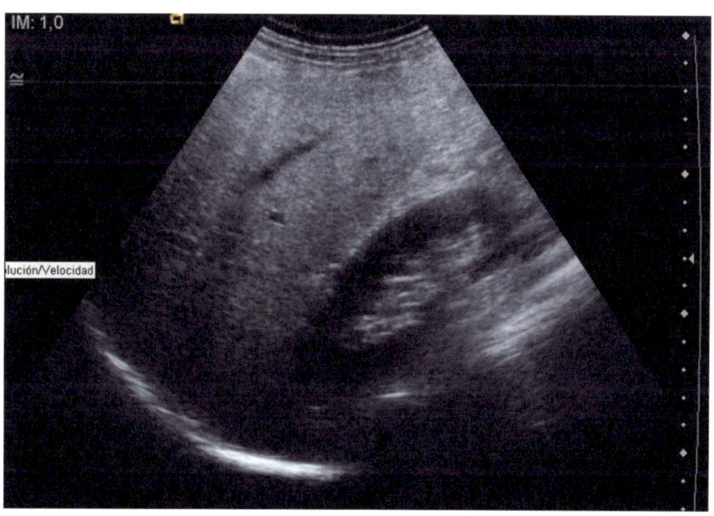

Figure 3.
Heterogeneous liver in a patient with AUD admitted for hospital detoxification.

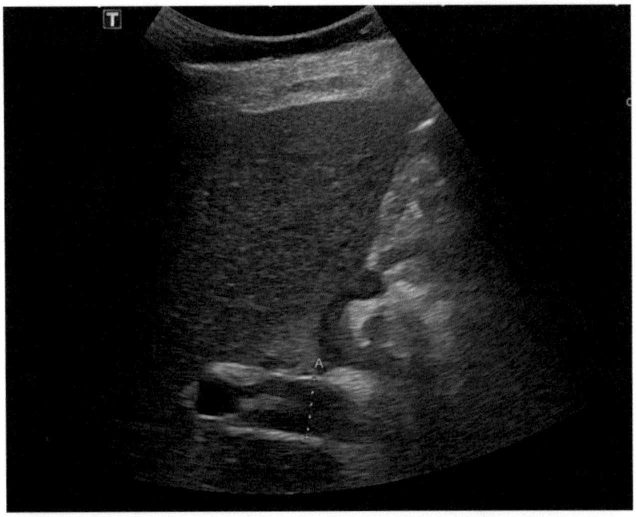

Figure 4.
Cirrhosis of the liver with an enlarged portal vein, consistent with portal hypertension.

bluntness of the edge, coarseness of parenchyma, nodularity of the surface, size of the lymph nodes around the hepatic artery, irregularity and narrowness of the inferior vena cava, portal vein velocity and caliber, and spleen size [28].

Figure 3 shows a heterogeneous liver in a 45-year-old patient with alcohol-related liver disease, and **Figure 4** shows an ultrasound of a 50-year-old patient with AUD and alcohol-related cirrhosis of the liver, as well as an enlarged portal vein, consistent with portal hypertension.

5. Use of liver ultrasound in patients with AUD: current evidence

Evidence about the use of liver ultrasounds to detect underlying liver disease in patients with AUD is scarce and includes a Cochrane systematic review and a recently published study by our group.

5.1 Cochrane systematic review

A Cochrane review published in 2016 stated that there was a need for studies of adequate sample size to study the efficacy of liver ultrasound in alcohol-related liver disease [39], as the review could only include two studies that aimed to assess alcohol-related liver cirrhosis with liver ultrasound [39].

The first study was published by French researchers in 1985 and included 126 alcoholic patients who underwent liver ultrasound [40]. Of those, a hundred patients also underwent liver biopsy. The mean age of participants was 55.6 years. In that study, the main ultrasound findings were as follows: 100 patients (78%) presented hepatomegaly, 59 (46%) presented heterogeneous liver, 44 (34%) presented portal hypertension, and 82 (64%) presented liver cirrhosis. In those who underwent liver biopsy, liver cirrhosis was confirmed in 72 participants, so ultrasound had a 81% sensitivity and 79% specificity for the detection of liver cirrhosis [40].

The second study was performed in Korea and published in 2013. It included 230 patients (81% male) who underwent abdominal ultrasound and liver elastography prior to liver biopsy [41]. The mean age of the study population was 50.4 years; 199 patients (86.5%) and 170 (74%) presented an ultrasound that was suggestive of heterogeneous liver and liver cirrhosis, respectively. Liver cirrhosis was confirmed in 111 participants; therefore, ultrasound had a 94% sensitivity and 49% specificity for the detection of liver cirrhosis [41].

Due to differences in the selection criteria and the small number of patients included in both studies, the systematic review could reach no conclusion around the usefulness of liver ultrasound to detect underlying liver cirrhosis in patients with alcohol use [39].

5.2 Ultrasound findings of liver damage in a series of AUD patients consecutively admitted for hospital detoxification

We recently published a cross-sectional study of the use of abdominal ultrasound in 301 patients with AUD without overt liver disease that were admitted for hospital detoxification [17].

In that study, clinical and laboratory parameters were obtained at admission, and an abdominal ultrasound was performed on the third day of admission. Abdominal ultrasound was used to identify steatosis, hepatomegaly, heterogeneous liver, and portal hypertension. Portal hypertension was defined as having any of the following abnormalities: splenomegaly, enlarged portal vein, ascites, and/or abnormal portal vein flow.

For the purpose of the analysis, we defined analytical liver injury (ALI) as at least two of the following abnormalities: aspartate aminotransferase (AST) levels $\geq 74 < 300$ U/L, AST/alanine aminotransferase (ALT) ratio >2, and total bilirubin>1.2 mg/dL. Advanced liver fibrosis (ALF) was measured with the FIB-4 (a noninvasive index for the detection of liver fibrosis) [42], and was defined as a FIB-4 score ≥ 3.25.

We wanted to study bivariate associations of ultrasound abnormalities with three commonly observed conditions, hepatitis C virus infection (HCV), ALI, and ALF. We also used logistic regression to see if any of those three conditions predicted the presence of two or more ultrasound abnormalities.

In brief, 80% of the participants were male, with a median age of 46 years (Interquartile range [IQR]: 39–51 years) and had an alcohol consumption of 180 g/day upon admission (IQR: 120–201 g). The prevalence of HCV was 21.2%; AST and ALT serum levels were 42 U/L (IQR: 23–78 U/L) and 35 U/L (IQR: 19–60 U/L), respectively; 16% of patients had ALI and 24% ALF. Ultrasound findings in the study population were as follows: 57.2% steatosis, 49.5% hepatomegaly, 17% heterogeneous liver, and 16% portal hypertension. Of note, 77% had at least one ultrasound abnormality, and 45% had ≥2.

In logistic regression analyses, ALI and ALF were associated with having ≥2 ultrasound abnormalities [Odds Ratio (OR) (95% Confidence Interval [CI]): 5.2 (2.1–12.8), $p < 0.01$ and 4.7 (2.2–9.7), $p < 0.01$, respectively], while HCV infection was not (we performed a multivariate regression model for each of the three potential predictors) [17].

Most patients with only one ultrasound abnormality had hepatomegaly or mild to moderate steatosis, both of which represent morphologic changes that are potentially reversible with alcohol cessation. Therefore, we believe that implementation of abdominal ultrasound in the regular care of patients seeking AUD treatment might be helpful for making clinical decisions and determining therapeutic interventions.

In fact, ultrasound abnormalities were very common in this series of patients, even in patients without HCV, ALI, and ALF, as only 31% of patients in that group had a totally normal abdominal ultrasound. In this regard, we believe that the use of ultrasound to detect early stages of liver disease may promote alcohol cessation, what might have a tremendous impact on the natural history of alcohol-related liver cirrhosis, especially in patients that present earlier stages of the disease [17]. As previously described by other researchers, sharing findings that might impact negatively the prognosis with patients may also be associated with a decrease in unhealthy drinking [18]. Upon publication of this study, a literature search did not identify any large ultrasound study of AUD patients with compensated liver disease [17].

5.3 Hepatocellular carcinoma surveillance

As mentioned before, hepatocellular carcinoma is the last stage of alcohol-related liver disease, with an annual incidence of 2.9% in patients that already harbor liver cirrhosis [10]. It entails a very poor prognosis if not detected at the earliest possible stage [43]. This is the reason why all patients with alcohol-related cirrhosis should be included in hepatocellular carcinoma surveillance programs that typically consist of an abdominal ultrasound every 6 months [10].

However, periodical surveillance is not optimal in clinical practice, as surveillance is missed by one-third of patients and the interval between screening ultrasounds is often greater than 6 months [10]. In fact, less than 30% of hepatocellular carcinomas diagnosed in Europe and the USA are detected by surveillance [10, 44]. In addition, patients with alcohol-related liver cirrhosis are more likely to have deficient surveillance than those with HCV infection [43, 45].

In our series of 301 patients with AUD that underwent liver ultrasound, 15 (4.9%) had space occupying lesions; most of those lesions were hepatic hemangiomas, but hepatocellular carcinoma was diagnosed in 2 patients [17].

Figure 5 shows a liver nodule, suggestive of hepatocellular carcinoma over a cirrhotic liver in a 52-year-old woman with AUD and untreated chronic HCV.

5.4 Other potential uses of abdominal ultrasound in patients with AUD

Beyond the early detection of liver steatosis or liver cirrhosis, abdominal ultrasound might be useful for the detection of other forms of liver disease that may coexist with alcohol-related liver disease.

Alcohol use is common in patients with other forms of liver disease, and even alcohol use that would be considered moderate can be detrimental in these

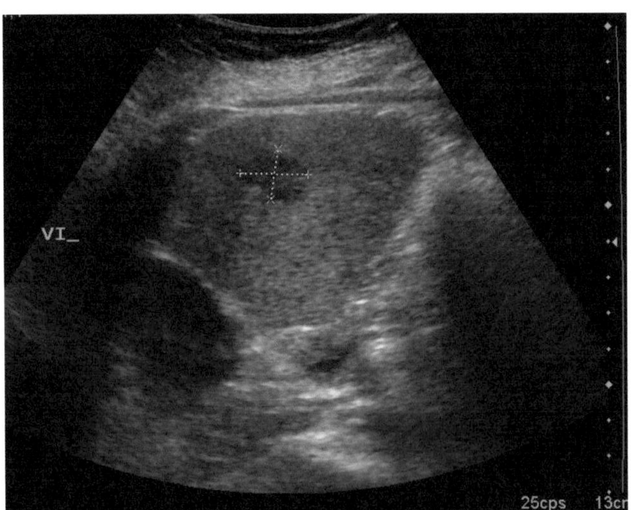

Figure 5.
A liver nodule, suggestive of hepatocellular carcinoma over a cirrhotic liver in a 52-year-old woman with AUD and untreated chronic hepatitis C virus infection.

situations [46, 47]. In fact, alcohol use is a cofactor for the progression of liver disease in patients with HCV, hepatitis B virus infection (HBV), nonalcoholic fatty liver disease, and hemochromatosis, among others. It is important to note that an arbitrary threshold of a daily alcohol intake of 30 grams for men and 20 grams for women is used to differentiate between alcohol-related liver damage and damage due to other etiologies [2]. However, with the current epidemic of overweight and obesity in Western societies, alcohol-related liver disease and nonalcoholic liver steatosis often coexist in the same patient [48]. In fact, in our cohort of patients with AUD that underwent abdominal ultrasound, the median body mass index was 24.7 kg/m^2, that is, a significant amount of patients were overweight [17].

In addition, the performance of abdominal ultrasound can detect less prevalent forms of liver disease, like vascular diseases (Budd-Chiari syndrome, hepatic vein congestion, and noncirrhotic portal hypertension) as well as other parenchymatous diseases.

6. Other noninvasive procedures used to detect liver steatosis in patients with AUD

Controlled attenuation parameter (CAP) is a noninvasive tool to detect liver steatosis that measures ultrasound attenuation when trespassing fatty liver tissue [49]. CAP software is incorporated into the transient elastography equipment, thus facilitating the bedside estimation of both liver steatosis and liver fibrosis [14].

In a recent individual patient data meta-analysis that included 2, 735 cases with both liver biopsy and CAP, cutoffs for moderate and severe liver steatosis were defined, with a diagnostic accuracy between 0.65 and 0.90 [50]. Patients included in that meta-analysis had mainly HBV (37%) and HCV (36%), or nonalcoholic fatty liver disease (20%), while patients with alcohol-related liver disease were underrepresented [50]. Given that all patients included in the meta-analysis harbored liver diseases that are strongly associated with liver fibrosis, there is a need for further validation of those cutoffs in a healthier population [51].

Another study by Thiele and colleagues published in 2018 that included 562 patients with alcohol-related liver steatosis found that CAP above 290 dB/m ruled in any steatosis with 88% specificity and 92% positive predictive value, while CAP below 220 dB/m ruled out steatosis with 90% sensitivity, but 62% negative predictive value [52]. Researchers concluded that CAP had a good diagnostic accuracy for diagnosing severe alcoholic liver steatosis and could be used to rule in any steatosis. The study also included a cohort of patients who were admitted for alcohol detoxification and found that CAP rapidly declined in nonobese patients [52]. This finding speaks to the double-hit model of alcohol use and obesity in a significant proportion of patients commonly seen in clinical practice [53].

7. Alternative noninvasive methods to detect liver fibrosis in patients with AUD

7.1 Transient elastography

Transient elastography has also been used for analyzing liver injury in patients with AUD. A study found elastography provided an assessment of fibrosis that was comparable to liver biopsy [16]. Other authors, however, have expressed concerns that alcohol-related steatohepatitis may distort results, leading to overestimation of liver fibrosis in this population [54], especially in patients who maintain abstinence from alcohol, as liver stiffness seems to dramatically decrease with cessation of alcohol use [55].

A systematic review and meta-analysis published in 2016 that included 14 different studies suggested that transient elastography was a good method to exclude the presence of liver cirrhosis or advanced liver cirrhosis but advised that caution should be needed when using the same cutoffs described for viral hepatitis in other forms of liver disease [56].

A recently published individual patient data meta-analysis that included 1026 patients suggested that cutoffs for transient elastography should be higher, especially in patients with elevated AST and/or bilirubin, suggestive of active alcoholic hepatitis [57].

Therefore, transient elastography is a promising tool, but it is mainly used in European countries in specialty clinics or teaching institutions [14]. In other countries its use is limited because of budget constraints or because it is only approved for research purposes.

7.2 Noninvasive laboratory-driven indices

There are several noninvasive indices to estimate liver fibrosis that are derived from laboratory parameters routinely used in clinical practice, including AST, ALT, and platelet count.

Among those, the most widely used are the FIB-4 [42], and the AST/platelet ratio index (APRI) [58], which have been validated against the gold standard of liver biopsy in HCV-monoinfected patients as well as HCV- and HIV-coinfected patients [59–61]. These indices perform better for detecting either the absence of liver fibrosis or the presence of advanced liver fibrosis [42, 58]. However, clinical experience using these markers in patients with AUD is somewhat limited [62]. In fact, some researchers have expressed concerns because of potential overestimation of liver fibrosis when using these noninvasive indices in alcohol-related liver disease [62, 63].

In a series of patients with HIV and/or HCV infection, results around the ability of noninvasive indices to capture the impact of alcohol and liver fibrosis have been mixed, probably because of the different methods used to describe alcohol intake and other characteristics of the study population. A cross-sectional study in an urban cohort of HIV-infected individuals in Baltimore (USA) revealed that heavy alcohol use was associated with advanced liver fibrosis measured using the APRI score [64]. In that same study, when patients were stratified by HCV infection, high APRI score was associated with hazardous alcohol use only among patients without HCV infection [64]. In a cohort of HIV-infected women, Blackard and colleagues demonstrated that alcohol use was not associated with FIB-4 values among those with HCV-/HIV-coinfected women [65].

In a cohort of Boston HIV-infected patients with alcohol problems, lifetime alcohol consumption was not associated with the presence of advanced liver fibrosis (FIB-4 $\geq$ 3.25) [66, 67]. Another study performed in the Veterans Aging Cohort Study (VACS) reported greater risks of advanced liver fibrosis (measured with FIB-4) among HCV-/HIV-coinfected patients who exhibited any level of alcohol consumption or who had alcohol-related diagnoses [68].

Despite these somewhat discordant results, noninvasive markers of liver fibrosis have been widely used in populations with alcohol or other substance use disorders that are unlikely to undergo a liver biopsy [67, 69]. Besides, those noninvasive indices have been able to predict midterm mortality in epidemiological studies [69, 70]. A rather innovative approach is the combination of noninvasive indices and transient elastography, so as to better characterize patients in the intermediate range of FIB-4 values (1.45–3.25) [71].

8. Conclusions

Abdominal ultrasound is a cheap and easily available noninvasive method that could be useful as a first-line screening to assess underlying liver disease in patients with excessive alcohol intake. For patients that need further assessment, transient elastography and CAP, if available, might be helpful in defining the extent and magnitude of alcohol-related liver disease.

Acknowledgements

The research was partially funded by the Ministry of Economy and Competitiveness; Institute of Health Carlos III (RETICS RD16/0017/0003, grant PI17/00174, and Rio Hortega Program CM17/022), Spain; and European Fund for Regional Development (FEDER); Ministry of Health, Social Services and Equality, and National Plan on Drugs (grants 2015/027 and 2018/020), Spain; Gilead Fellowship Program, Gilead Sciences (grant GLD17/00187); Health Department Intensification Program (grant SLT006/17/00107) and Consolidated Research Group (grant 2017-SGR-316), Autonomous of Catalonia, Spain.

Conflict of interest

The authors report no conflict of interest.

Author details

Daniel Fuster[1]*, Xavier Garcia-Calvo[1], Paola Zuluaga[1], Inmaculada Rivas[2], Arantza Sanvisens[1], Jordi Tor[1] and Robert Muga[1]

1 Internal Medicine Service, Hospital Universitari Germans Trias i Pujol, Universitat Autònoma de Barcelona, Badalona, Spain

2 Municipal Centre for Substance Abuse Treatment (Centro Delta), Badalona Serveis Assistencials, Badalona, Spain

*Address all correspondence to: dfuster.germanstrias@gencat.cat

References

[1] Griswold MG, Fullman N, Hawley C, et al. Alcohol use and burden for 195 countries and territories, 1990-2016: A systematic analysis for the global burden of disease study 2016. Lancet. 2018;**392**(10152):1015-1035. DOI: 10.1016/S0140-6736(18)31310-2

[2] Fuster D, Samet JH. Alcohol use in patients with chronic liver disease. The New England Journal of Medicine. 2018;**379**(26):2577-2579. DOI: 10.1056/NEJMc1814129

[3] Rehm J, Samokhvalov AV, Shield KD. Global burden of alcoholic liver diseases. Journal of Hepatology. 2013;**59**(1):160-168. DOI: 10.1016/j.jhep.2013.03.007

[4] Jinjuvadia R, Liangpunsakul S. Translational research and evolving alcoholic hepatitis treatment consortium. Trends in alcoholic hepatitis-related hospitalizations, financial burden, and mortality in the United States. Journal of Clinical Gastroenterology. 2015;**49**(6):506-511. DOI: 10.1097/MCG.0000000000000161

[5] Williams R, Aspinall R, Bellis M, et al. Addressing liver disease in the UK: A blueprint for attaining excellence in health care and reducing premature mortality from lifestyle issues of excess consumption of alcohol, obesity, and viral hepatitis. Lancet. 2014;**384**(9958):1953-1997. DOI: 10.1016/S0140-6736(14)61838-9

[6] Stein E, Cruz-Lemini M, Altamirano J, et al. Heavy daily alcohol intake at the population level predicts the weight of alcohol in cirrhosis burden worldwide. Journal of Hepatology. 2016;**65**(5):998-1005. DOI: 10.1016/j.jhep.2016.06.018

[7] Bataller R, Arteel GE, Moreno C, Shah V. Alcohol-related liver disease: Time for action. Journal of Hepatology. 2019;**70**(2):221-222. DOI: 10.1016/j.jhep.2018.12.007

[8] Roson B, Monte R, Gamallo R, et al. Prevalence and routine assessment of unhealthy alcohol use in hospitalized patients. European Journal of Internal Medicine. 2010;**21**(5):458-464. DOI: 10.1016/j.ejim.2010.04.006; 1

[9] Seitz HK, Bataller R, Cortez-Pinto H, et al. Alcoholic liver disease. Nature Reviews. Disease Primers. 2018;**4**(1):16. DOI: 10.1038/s41572-018-0014-7

[10] Ganne-Carrié N, Nahon P. Hepatocellular carcinoma in the setting of alcohol-related liver disease. Journal of Hepatology. 2019;**70**(2):284-293. DOI: 10.1016/j.jhep.2018.10.008

[11] Lackner C, Tiniakos D. Fibrosis and alcohol-related liver disease. Journal of Hepatology. 2019;**70**(2):294-304. DOI: 10.1016/j.jhep.2018.12.003

[12] Mathurin P, Moreno C, Samuel D, et al. Early liver transplantation for severe alcoholic hepatitis. The New England Journal of Medicine. 2011;**365**(19):1790-1800. DOI: 10.1056/NEJMoa1105703

[13] Ratib S, Fleming KM, Crooks CJ, Walker AJ, West J. Causes of death in people with liver cirrhosis in England compared with the general population: A population-based cohort study. The American Journal of Gastroenterology. 2015;**110**(8):1149-1158. DOI: 10.1038/ajg.2015.191

[14] Moreno C, Mueller S, Szabo G. Non-invasive diagnosis and biomarkers in alcohol-related liver disease. Journal of Hepatology. 2019;**70**(2):273-283. DOI: 10.1016/j.jhep.2018.11.025

[15] Ratziu V, Bellentani S, Cortez-Pinto H, Day C, Marchesini G. A position statement on NAFLD/NASH based

on the EASL 2009 special conference. Journal of Hepatology. 2010;**53**(2): 372-384. DOI: 10.1016/j.jhep.2010.04.008

[16] Thiele M, Detlefsen S, Sevelsted Møller L, et al. Transient and 2-dimensional shear-wave elastography provide comparable assessment of alcoholic liver fibrosis and cirrhosis. Gastroenterology. 2016;**150**(1):123-133. DOI: 10.1053/j.gastro.2015.09.040

[17] Fuster D, Garcia-Calvo X, Zuluaga P, et al. Ultrasound findings of liver damage in a series of patients consecutively admitted for treatment of alcohol use disorder. Drug and Alcohol Dependence. 2018;**190**:195-199. DOI: 10.1016/j.drugalcdep.2018.06.012

[18] Tsui JI, Saitz R, Cheng DM, et al. Awareness of hepatitis C diagnosis is associated with less alcohol use among persons co-infected with HIV. Journal of General Internal Medicine. 2007;**22**(6):822-825. DOI: 10.1007/s11606-007-0147-y

[19] Saunders JB, Aasland OG, Babor TF, de la Fuente JR, Grant M. Development of the alcohol use disorders identification test (AUDIT): WHO collaborative project on early detection of persons with harmful alcohol consumption--II. Addiction. 1993;**88**(6):791-804

[20] American Psychiatric Association. Diagnostic and Statistical Manual of Mental Disorders. 4th ed. (DSM IV-TR) ed. Washington DC: Government Printing Office; 2000

[21] Diagnostic and Statistical Manual of Mental Disorders, DSM-5. Washington DC: American Psychiatric Association, Government Printing Office; 2013

[22] O'Shea RS, Dasarathy S, McCullough AJ. Practice guideline Committee of the American Association for the study of liver, practice parameters Committee of the American College of gastroenterology. Alcoholic liver disease. Hepatology. 2010;**51**(1):307-328. DOI: 10.1002/hep.23258

[23] Thursz M, Gual A, Lackner C, et al. EASL clinical practice guidelines: Management of alcohol-related liver disease. Journal of Hepatology. 2018;**69**(1):154-181. DOI: 10.1016/j.jhep.2018.03.018

[24] Bush K, Kivlahan DR, McDonell MB, Fihn SD, Bradley KA. The AUDIT alcohol consumption questions (AUDIT-C): An effective brief screening test for problem drinking. Ambulatory care quality improvement project (ACQUIP). Alcohol Use Disorders Identification Test. Archives of Internal Medicine. 1998;**158**(16):1789-1795

[25] Smith PC, Schmidt SM, Allensworth-Davies D, Saitz R. A single-question screening test for drug use in primary care. Archives of Internal Medicine. 2010;**170**(13):1155-1160. DOI: 10.1001/archinternmed.2010.140

[26] Kratzer W, Fritz V, Mason RA, Haenle MM, Kaechele V, Roemerstein Study Group. Factors affecting liver size: A sonographic survey of 2080 subjects. Journal of Ultrasound in Medicine. 2003;**22**(11):1155-1161

[27] Strauss S, Gavish E, Gottlieb P, Katsnelson L. Interobserver and intraobserver variability in the sonographic assessment of fatty liver. AJR. American Journal of Roentgenology. 2007;**189**(6):W320-W323. DOI: 10.2214/AJR.07.2123

[28] American College of Radiology. Practice Parameter for the Performance of an Ultrasound Examination of the Abdomen and/or Retroperitoneum. 2018. Available at: https://www.acr.org/Quality-Safety/Standards-uidelines/media/ACR/Documents/PGTS/

guidelines/US_Abdomen_Retro.pdf [Accessed: December 12, 2019]

[29] Kim MY, Jeong WK, Baik SK. Invasive and non-invasive diagnosis of cirrhosis and portal hypertension. World Journal of Gastroenterology. 2014;**20**(15):4300. DOI: 10.3748/wjg.v20.i15.4300

[30] Kruskal JB, Newman PA, Sammons LG, Kane RA. Optimizing Doppler and color flow US: Application to hepatic sonography. Radiographics. 2004;**24**(3):657-675. DOI: 10.1148/rg.243035139

[31] Reinhold C, Hammers L, Taylor CR, Quedens-Case CL, Holland CK, Taylor KJ. Characterization of focal hepatic lesions with duplex sonography: Findings in 198 patients. AJR. American Journal of Roentgenology. 1995;**164**(5):1131-1135. DOI: 10.2214/ajr.164.5.7717219

[32] Schwenzer NF, Springer F, Schraml C, Stefan N, Machann J, Schick F. Non-invasive assessment and quantification of liver steatosis by ultrasound, computed tomography and magnetic resonance. Journal of Hepatology. 2009;**51**(3):433-445. DOI: 10.1016/j.jhep.2009.05.023

[33] Palmentieri B, de Sio I, La Mura V, et al. The role of bright liver echo pattern on ultrasound B-mode examination in the diagnosis of liver steatosis. Digestive and Liver Disease. 2006;**38**(7):485-489. DOI: 10.1016/j.dld.2006.03.021

[34] Taylor KJ, Gorelick FS, Rosenfield AT, Riely CA. Ultrasonography of alcoholic liver disease with histological correlation. Radiology. 1981;**141**(1):157-161. DOI: 10.1148/radiology.141.1.6270725

[35] Meek DR, Mills PR, Gray HW, Duncan JG, Russell RI, McKillop JH. A comparison of computed tomography, ultrasound and scintigraphy in the diagnosis of alcoholic liver disease. The British Journal of Radiology. 1984;**57**(673):23-27. DOI: 10.1259/0007-1285-57-673-23

[36] Hamaguchi M, Kojima T, Itoh Y, et al. The severity of ultrasonographic findings in nonalcoholic fatty liver disease reflects the metabolic syndrome and visceral fat accumulation. The American Journal of Gastroenterology. 2007;**102**(12):2708-2715. DOI: 10.1111/j.1572-0241.2007.01526.x

[37] Saverymuttu SH, Joseph AE, Maxwell JD. Ultrasound scanning in the detection of hepatic fibrosis and steatosis. British Medical Journal (Clinical Research Ed.). 1986;**292**(6512):13-15

[38] Mancini M, Prinster A, Annuzzi G, et al. Sonographic hepatic-renal ratio as indicator of hepatic steatosis: Comparison with 1H magnetic resonance spectroscopy. Metabolism. 2009;**58**(12):1724-1730. DOI: 10.1016/J.METABOL.2009.05.032

[39] Pavlov CS, Casazza G, Semenistaia M, et al. Ultrasonography for diagnosis of alcoholic cirrhosis in people with alcoholic liver disease. Cochrane Database of Systematic Reviews. 2016;**3**:CD011602. DOI: 10.1002/14651858.CD011602.pub2

[40] Richard P, Bonniaud P, Barthélémy C, et al. Value of ultrasonography in the diagnosis of cirrhoses. Prospective study of 128 patients. Journal de Radiologie;**66**(8-9):503-506. Available from: http://www.ncbi.nlm.nih.gov/pubmed/3912496 [Accessed: August 31, 2016]

[41] Moon KM, Kim G, Baik SK, et al. Ultrasonographic scoring system score versus liver stiffness measurement in prediction of cirrhosis. Clinical and Molecular Hepatology. 2013;**19**(4):389-398. DOI: 10.3350/cmh.2013.19.4.389

[42] Sterling RK, Lissen E, Clumeck N, et al. Development of a simple noninvasive index to predict significant fibrosis in patients with HIV/HCV coinfection. Hepatology. 2006;**43**(6):1317-1325. DOI: 10.1002/hep.21178

[43] Schütte K, Bornschein J, Kahl S, et al. Delayed diagnosis of HCC with chronic alcoholic liver disease. Liver Cancer. 2012;**1**(3-4):257-266. DOI: 10.1159/000343840

[44] Davila JA, Morgan RO, Richardson PA, Du XL, McGlynn KA, El-Serag HB. Use of surveillance for hepatocellular carcinoma among patients with cirrhosis in the United States. Hepatology. 2010;**52**(1):132-141. DOI: 10.1002/hep.23615

[45] Bucci L, Garuti F, Camelli V, et al. Comparison between alcohol- and hepatitis C virus-related hepatocellular carcinoma: Clinical presentation, treatment and outcome. Alimentary Pharmacology & Therapeutics. 2016;**43**(3):385-399. DOI: 10.1111/apt.13485

[46] Hutchinson SJ, Bird SM, Goldberg DJ. Influence of alcohol on the progression of hepatitis C virus infection: A meta-analysis. Clinical Gastroenterology and Hepatology. 2005;**3**(11):1150-1159

[47] Hagström H. Alcohol consumption in concomitant liver disease: How much is too much? Current Hepatology Reports. 2017;**16**(2):152-157. DOI: 10.1007/s11901-017-0343-0

[48] Ajmera VH, Terrault NA, Harrison SA. Is moderate alcohol use in nonalcoholic fatty liver disease good or bad? A critical review. Hepatology. 2017;**65**(6):2090-2099. DOI: 10.1002/hep.29055

[49] Sasso M, Beaugrand M, de Ledinghen V, et al. Controlled attenuation parameter (CAP): A novel VCTE™ guided ultrasonic attenuation measurement for the evaluation of hepatic steatosis: Preliminary study and validation in a cohort of patients with chronic liver disease from various causes. Ultrasound in Medicine & Biology. 2010;**36**(11):1825-1835. DOI: 10.1016/j.ultrasmedbio.2010.07.005

[50] Karlas T, Petroff D, Sasso M, et al. Individual patient data meta-analysis of controlled attenuation parameter (CAP) technology for assessing steatosis. Journal of Hepatology. 2017;**66**(5):1022-1030. DOI: 10.1016/j.jhep.2016.12.022

[51] Romero-Gómez M, Cortez-Pinto H. Detecting liver fat from viscoelasticity: How good is CAP in clinical practice? The need for universal cut-offs. Journal of Hepatology. 2017;**66**(5):886-887. DOI: 10.1016/J.JHEP.2017.01.029

[52] Thiele M, Rausch V, Fluhr G, et al. Controlled attenuation parameter and alcoholic hepatic steatosis: Diagnostic accuracy and role of alcohol detoxification. Journal of Hepatology. 2018;**68**(5):1025-1032. DOI: 10.1016/j.jhep.2017.12.029

[53] Bellentani S, Saccoccio G, Masutti F, et al. Prevalence of and risk factors for hepatic steatosis in northern Italy. Annals of Internal Medicine. 2000;**132**(2):112-117

[54] Mueller S, Englert S, Seitz HK, et al. Inflammation-adapted liver stiffness values for improved fibrosis staging in patients with hepatitis C virus and alcoholic liver disease. Liver International. 2015;**35**(12):2514-2521. DOI: 10.1111/liv.12904

[55] Gianni E, Forte P, Galli V, Razzolini G, Bardazzi G, Annese V. Prospective evaluation of liver stiffness using transient elastography in alcoholic patients following abstinence. Alcohol

and Alcoholism. 2017;**52**(1):42-47. DOI: 10.1093/alcalc/agw053

[56] Pavlov CS, Casazza G, Nikolova D, Tsochatzis E, Gluud C. Systematic review with meta-analysis: Diagnostic accuracy of transient elastography for staging of fibrosis in people with alcoholic liver disease. Alimentary Pharmacology & Therapeutics. 2016;**43**(5):575-585. DOI: 10.1111/apt.13524

[57] Nguyen-Khac E, Thiele M, Voican C,et al. Non-invasive diagnosis of liver fibrosis in patients with alcohol-related liver disease by transient elastography: An individual patient data meta-analysis. The Lancet Gastroenterology & Hepatology. 2018;**3**(9):614-625. DOI: 10.1016/S2468-1253(18)30124-9

[58] Wai CT, Greenson JK, Fontana RJ, et al. A simple noninvasive index can predict both significant fibrosis and cirrhosis in patients with chronic hepatitis C. Hepatology. 2003;**38**(2):518-526. DOI: 10.1053/jhep.2003.50346

[59] Nunes D, Fleming C, Offner G, et al. HIV infection does not affect the performance of noninvasive markers of fibrosis for the diagnosis of hepatitis C virus-related liver disease. Journal of Acquired Immune Deficiency Syndromes. 2005;**40**(5):538-544

[60] Loko MA, Castera L, Dabis F, et al. Validation and comparison of simple noninvasive indexes for predicting liver fibrosis in HIV-HCV-coinfected patients: ANRS CO3 Aquitaine cohort. The American Journal of Gastroenterology. 2008;**103**(8):1973-1980. DOI: 10.1111/j.1572-0241.2008.01954.x

[61] Vallet-Pichard A, Mallet V, Nalpas B, et al. FIB-4: An inexpensive and accurate marker of fibrosis in HCV infection. Comparison with liver biopsy and fibrotest. Hepatology. 2007;**46**(1):32-36. DOI: 10.1002/hep.21669

[62] Lieber CS, Weiss DG, Morgan TR, Paronetto F. Aspartate aminotransferase to platelet ratio index in patients with alcoholic liver fibrosis. The American Journal of Gastroenterology. 2006;**101**(7):1500-1508. DOI: 10.1111/j.1572-0241.2006.00610.x

[63] Trabut J-B, Thépot V, Terris B, Sogni P, Nalpas B, Pol S. Prognosis assessment of alcoholic liver disease: How and why? Presse Médicale. 2014;**43**(2):124-134. DOI: 10.1016/j.lpm.2013.04.016

[64] Chaudhry AA, Sulkowski MS, Chander G, Moore RD. Hazardous drinking is associated with an elevated aspartate aminotransferase to platelet ratio index in an urban HIV-infected clinical cohort. HIV Medicine. 2009;**10**(3):133-142. DOI: 10.1111/j.1468-1293.2008.00662.x

[65] Blackard JT, Welge JA, Taylor LE, et al. HIV mono-infection is associated with FIB-4 - a noninvasive index of liver fibrosis - in women. Clinical Infectious Diseases. 2011;**52**(5):674-680. DOI: 10.1093/cid/ciq199

[66] Skinner HA, Sheu WJ. Reliability of alcohol use indices. The lifetime drinking history and the MAST. Journal of Studies on Alcohol. 1982;**43**(11):1157-1170

[67] Fuster D, Tsui JI, Cheng DM, et al. Impact of lifetime alcohol use on liver fibrosis in a population of HIV-infected patients with and without hepatitis C coinfection. Alcoholism, Clinical and Experimental Research. 2013;**37**(9):1527-1535. DOI: 10.1111/acer.12129

[68] Lim JK, Tate JP, Fultz SL, et al. Relationship between alcohol use categories and noninvasive markers of advanced hepatic fibrosis in HIV-infected, chronic hepatitis

C virus-infected, and uninfected patients. Clinical Infectious Diseases. 2014;**58**(10):1449-1458. DOI: 10.1093/cid/ciu097

[69] Nunes D, Fleming C, Offner G, et al. Noninvasive markers of liver fibrosis are highly predictive of liver-related death in a cohort of HCV-infected individuals with and without HIV infection. The American Journal of Gastroenterology. 2010;**105**(6):1346-1353. DOI: 10.1038/ajg.2009.746

[70] Sanvisens A, Fuster D, Serra I, et al. Estimated liver fibrosis and its impact on all-cause mortality of HCV-monoinfected and HCV/HIV-coinfected drug users. Current HIV Research. 2011;**9**(4):256-262

[71] Gnatienko N, Freiberg MS, Blokhina E, et al. Design of a randomized controlled trial of zinc supplementation to improve markers of mortality and HIV disease progression in HIV-positive drinkers in St. Petersburg, Russia. HIV Clinical Trials. 2018;**19**(3):101-111. DOI: 10.1080/15284336.2018.1459344

Section 4

Kidneys Ultrasound

Chapter 4

The Kidney

Ercan Ayaz

Abstract

Ultrasound and conventional radiographs still remain the first-line radiological tools for most of the kidney disorders. Ultrasonographic image quality has been astonishingly improved in recent years with the development of technology and software algorithms. In line with these developments, ultrasound is not only the primary imaging modality for kidney anatomy and lesions, but also sufficient for definitive diagnosis and follow up for some lesions. The aim of this chapter is to focus on the areas that ultrasound is used primarily about the kidney. These topics include kidney anatomy, anatomic variants that mimic lesions, congenital diseases, kidney stones, nephrocalcinosis, most of the cystic diseases, and some solid lesions, infection, and trauma.

Keywords: kidney, ultrasound, renal cyst, kidney stone, nephrocalcinosis

1. Introduction

Major functions of the kidney are excreting metabolic waste products and maintaining homeostasis by regulating water, salt, and acid-base balance. The kidney is also an endocrine organ that secretes many hormones, including erythropoietin, renin, and prostaglandins. Ultrasound (US) represents the first-line radiologic imaging technique in the assessment of the kidney anatomy and various disorders. Imaging quality of US has greatly developed in recent years with the advances in the transducer, beam-former technology, and image processing software. Grayscale B-mode US, with the addition of tissue harmonic imaging and compound modes, and color Doppler US definitely provide a diagnostic clue in most renal abnormalities. US artifacts are extremely important in the US evaluation of the kidney because they must be differentiated by true images and may add valuable information in some lesions such as stone and cyst. US presents several advantages over the other imaging modalities including low financial cost, portability, availability, lack of restrictions in performing frequent serial examinations at short intervals, and absence of exposure to radiation or nuclear tracers.

In this chapter, grayscale US findings of normal kidney anatomy, anatomic variants, congenital anomalies, kidney stones, cystic and solid lesions, infections, and traumatic lesions have been discussed. Moreover, embryology and anatomy of the kidney have been explained along with the sonography technique briefly.

2. Embryology and anatomy

During the third week of the development of the human embryo, the urogenital apparatus derives from the intermediate mesoderm. The intermediate mesoderm

IntechOpen

initially divides into a set of small cell groups called nephrotomes in the cervical and thoracolumbar regions. These cell masses represent three different excretory sets: the pronephros, the mesonephros, and the metanephros. The pronephros is formed at the beginning of the fourth week and remains rudimentary. It is analogous to the kidney in primitive fishes. The mesonephros appears at the end of the fourth week and it is the first functioning unit until the development of metanephros at the ninth week [1]. It is analogous to the kidney of amphibians. Metanephros begins to be active in the 9–10th week [45]. After that time, it becomes a permanent kidney. Metanephros divided into two parts, which originate from different sources, called the metanephric mass and the metanpehric diverticulum. The metanephric mass derived from intermediate mesoderm and their cells give rise to nephrons which are the morphological functional units of the kidney. The metanephric diverticulum or ureteric bud develops from mesonephric duct, which constitutes collecting tubules, calices, renal pelvis, and ureter.

Initially, the permanent kidneys are located close to each other in the pelvis at the caudal end of the mesonephros and ventrally to the sacrum. With fetal growth, the kidneys progressively come to the retroperitoneum and move farther apart, while the abdomen and pelvis grow. At the end of the eighth week, the kidneys set themselves at the first four lumbar vertebral levels, just below the adrenal glands. This migration occurs not only by the caudal migration of the kidneys, but also the growth of the caudal part of the body away from the kidneys. The hilum of the kidney, which includes renal pelvis, vessels, and nerves, faces ventrally before migration; it rotates medially almost 90° during the ascent of kidney. In the ninth week, the renal pelvis is directed anteromedially [1].

During fetal life, the human kidney surface is lobulated which decreases gradually at the end of pregnancy but is still present in the kidneys of neonates. Lobulation disappears during infancy. The reason of the lobulation is the caliceal structure of the collecting system [45]. The buds of minor calices penetrate into the metanephric blastema and give rise to 13 trees of excretory ductules. Every minor calyx brings on a big glandular unit that consists of a medullar unit called Malpighi pyramid and a cortical unit which is separated from the others by interlobular sulci that causes lobulated surface of the kidney. Metanephric tissue penetrates between the pyramids, goes toward renal pelvis, and constitutes the Bertin column [1].

Primarily, fetal kidney derives blood supply, branches from the iliac artery. As the kidney ascends, it receives new branches from the abdominal aorta. Meanwhile, the branches from iliac artery undergo involution and disappear. Migration of the kidney ends at the ninth week, when the kidney takes tight contact with the suprarenal gland. Finally, the kidney receives the permanent renal arteries originating from the abdominal aorta. About 70% of people exhibit single renal artery to each kidney. On the other hand, two to four renal arteries are seen in 25% of adults [2]. The supernumerary arteries usually originate from the abdominal aorta above or below the main renal artery and follow it through the renal hilum. However, they may also enter the kidney from the superior and/or the inferior pole which is called polar artery. Inferior polar artery may cross anterior the ureter and occlude it, leading to hydronephrosis. It is important to recognize supernumerary arteries, since if an accessory artery is damaged or ligated, the region of the kidney supplied by it may undergo ischemia.

In the adult, each kidney is located in the retroperitoneum and measures approximately 10–12 cm long, 2–3 cm thick, and 3–5 cm wide and weighs 250–270 g [3]. The right kidney is located posterior to the inferior surface of the liver with peritoneal interposition, and lateral to the second portion of the duodenum without any peritoneal interposition since the second portion of the duodenum is retroperitoneal. The left kidney lies posterior to the pancreatic tail, the stomach, the ligament of Treitz, and posterior medial to the spleen.

The volume of the right kidney is smaller than that of the left kidney, possibly due to limited potential space for the right kidney (large volume of liver in the right upper quadrant) or relatively increased left renal flow (left kidney is closer to aorta and left renal artery is shorter than right renal artery) [4].

The kidney is a bean shaped organ with a smooth, regular border. Renal hilum is located at the medial surface of the kidney and continues with a central cavity called renal sinus. Renal sinus contains the major branches of the renal artery, major tributaries of the renal vein, and the collecting system [5]. The background of renal pelvis is composed of fat tissue. Renal pelvis is generally located posterior to the vessels. The kidney is covered by a renal capsule which is composed of an inner fibrous layer and an outer perinephric adipose layer. Renal cortex is the outer part of the kidney between fibrous renal capsule and the renal medulla. It has a smooth outer contour with a number of projections (columns of Bertin) extending between the Malpighi pyramids. Renal medulla is the inner part of the kidney consisting of a number of 8–18 cone shaped sections, known as renal pyramids. The inner tip of each renal pyramid is called renal papilla where the urine drains into the renal pelvis. The renal pelvis extrudes from the kidney anteromedially and continues as the ureter. The left kidney is usually located 1–2 cm higher than the right kidney and in supine position; right renal pelvis is usually located at the level of the second lumbar vertebra [6].

Renal pyramids are hypoechoic relative to the cortex in the adult kidney which allows demonstrating both structures in ultrasound. The renal cortex should be hypo- or isoechoic relative to the adjacent liver or spleen in most of the normal adults. Hyperechoic renal cortex showed a specificity of 96%and a positive predictive value of 67% for detecting abnormal renal function, but with a poor sensitivity (20%) [7]. However, in neonates, renal cortex is iso- or hyperechoic relative to liver and spleen parenchyma and pyramids are more prominent. Even in premature infants, cortical hyperechogenicity is more prominent [8]. However, an excessive increased renal echogenicity in newborns may also be due to infantile polycystic kidney disease, hemolytic-uremic syndrome, or renal vein thrombosis [8]. Within the range of 2–6 months, the kidneys become gradually less echogenic than the liver and assume the features of the adult kidney between 6 and 24 months of life [3].

There are some variations that affect the border and cortex of the kidney such as junctional parenchymal defect, fetal lobulations, dromedary hump, and hypertrophied column of Bertin (HCB) (**Figure 1**). HCB is an unresorbed polar parenchyma from one or both of the two subdivisions of kidneys that combine to form the normal kidney [9]. HCB is generally located at the junction of the upper and middle thirds of the kidney and contain renal cortex which extends to the renal sinus. HCB also contains adjacent renal pyramids and usually measures less than 3 cm [10]. Sometimes, echogenicity of the HCBs is different from the adjacent renal cortex due to alterations in tissue orientation, which result in different acoustic reflectivity [9]. It may be challenging to differentiate a small, avascular tumor from an HCB, and occasionally contrast enhanced computed tomography (CT) may be necessary to differentiate them.

Junctional parenchymal defects occur at the site of two parenchymal masses called ranunculi which constitute the normal kidney. It is a horizontally oriented linear echogenicity most often located anterior and superiorly and traced medially into the renal sinus.

Dromedary hump is a prominent bulging on the superolateral aspect of the left kidney. It is believed to arise secondary to compression of the upper pole of the left kidney by the spleen during development. The normal nature of this finding is appreciated by the constant thickness of the bulging renal cortex over the underlying renal calyces.

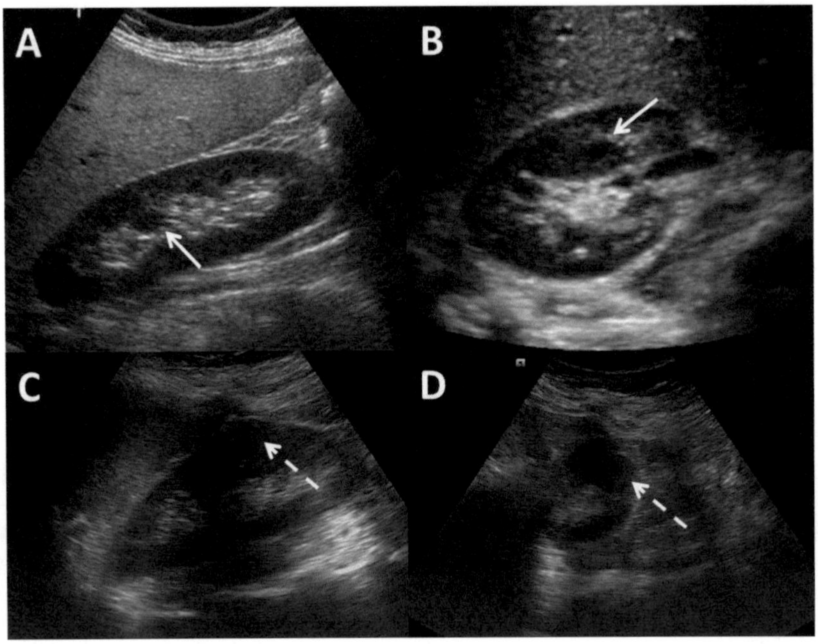

Figure 1.
Congenital variations of the kidney. On sagittal (A) and transverse (B) section of the kidney, hypertrophied column of Bertini (arrow) is seen as a hypoechoic cortical extension to the renal sinus. Sagittal (C) and transverse (D) section of another kidney reveals cortical bulging (dashed arrow) on the superolateral aspect, adjacent to the spleen termed as "dromedary hump".

3. Sonography technique

Before the examination, the adult patients should fast for a minimum of 6 hours before the examination to avoid extensive bowel gas. Convex-array US transducers (with a frequency of 2–5 MHz in adults and 5–8 MHz in pediatric patients) are usually preferred for the US scanning of the kidney. In newborns and infants, even in children, liner US transducers with higher frequency (8–12 MHz) should be additionally employed for better evaluation of cortex and medulla. Tissue harmonic imaging and compound imaging may often be useful for increasing lesion conspicuity and decreasing artifacts [11].

Optimal patient positioning depends on patient habitus, but supine and lateral decubitus positions are often sufficient; while the breath-hold technique is frequently necessary to obtain a complete examination of the renal parenchyma. If there is bowel gas superposition on subcostal view, intercostal window can be used to display kidneys on both sides. The kidneys should be evaluated in the transverse and coronal plane from the superior tip to the inferior [11].

4. Congenital anomalies

Ectopic kidneys are generally located at the pelvis (**Figure 2B**); however, it can be rarely located in the thorax. Crossed renal ectopia is defined as the presence of both kidneys in the same side of the body. The ectopic kidney is fused to the normal kidney in 85–90% of cases called crossed fused ectopy [12]. The upper pole of the ectopic kidney is commonly fused to the lower pole of the normal kidney. Fusion of the kidneys limits the ascent while developments, and thus, both kidneys are located caudally.

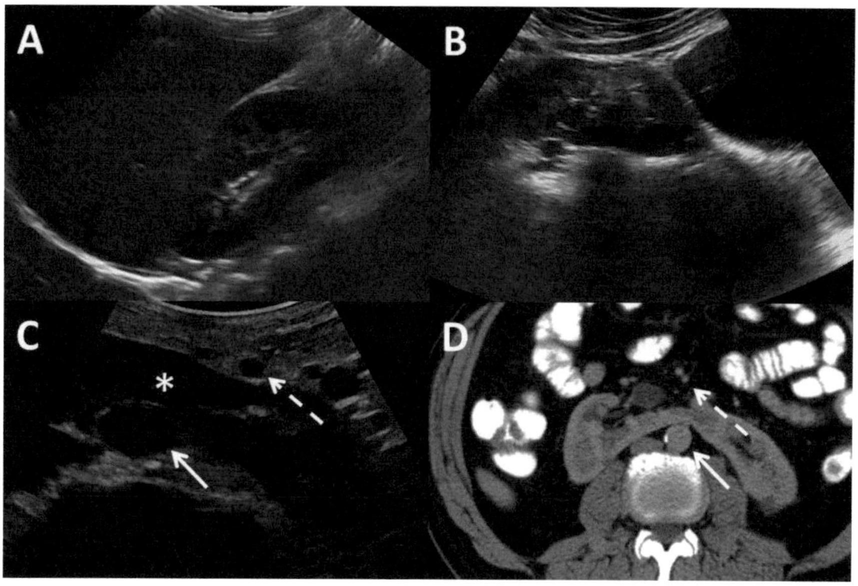

Figure 2.
Congenital anomalies of the kidney. Normal kidney is located inferomedially adjacent to the liver (A). An example of a right ectopic kidney located adjacent to the bladder (B). Ultrasound (C) and computed tomography (D) image of a horseshoe kidney reveals that right and left kidney fused from lower poles at the midline (asterix) from lower poles (asterix) and located between abdominal aorta (arrow) and inferior mesenteric artery (dashed arrow).

Horseshoe kidney is the fusion of the both metanephrogenic blastema from the lower poles prior to migration cranially. Isthmus may compose of either functioning renal cortex or fibrous tissue. The horseshoe kidney is more prone to infection and stone formation due to abnormal rotation of renal pelvis and ureteropelvic junction obstruction. On ultrasound, the horseshoe kidney is located more caudal than usual location and lower poles project inferomedially. Renal isthmus can be seen in the lower abdomen crossing the midline anterior to the aorta (**Figure 2C,D**).

Ureteropelvic junction (UPJ) obstruction is a common anomaly with a male preponderance and the left kidney suffers twice as frequently as the right kidney [13]. Patients with UPJ obstruction have an increased incidence of multicystic dysplastic kidney and renal agenesis of the other kidney. On ultrasound, marked hydronephrosis is present proximal to the level of UPJ obstruction along with normal caliber of the ureter. If long standing, renal parenchymal atrophy accompanies severe dilatation of the renal pelvis.

5. Nephrolithiasis and nephrocalcinosis

Nephrolithiasis is termed as calcification within the collecting system, bladder, ureter, and calyceal system, while nephrocalcinosis is defined as the deposition of calcium salts in the renal parenchyma.

Nephrolithiasis is a common disease with a prevalence of 2–3% in general population and 1.8/10,000 of hospital admissions [14, 15]. If we look at different regions of the world more closely, estimated prevalence is at 20.1% in Saudi Arabia, 1–5% in Asia, 5–9% in Europe, and 12–13% in Canada and North America [16]. White men who are in their fourth and fifth decade are affected most commonly [17]. A majority of the patients are present with acute, severe flank pain when a kidney stone becomes impacted in the ureter due to obstruction, dysuria, strangury, and hematuria. Almost 70% of kidney stones are composed of calcium, and patients with calcium stones are more prone to further stone formation within 7 years [16].

Multiple predisposing factors have been identified for nephrolithiasis including metabolic diseases such as cystinuria (autosomal recessive) and hyperoxaluria, inherited conditions (polycystic kidney disease, renal tubular acidosis, hyperparathyroidism, and hypercalciuria), medications (triamterene, sulfonamides, carbonic anhydrase inhibitors, indinavir, acetazolamide, and corticosteroids), low urine volume, hypercalciuria (hyperparathyroidism and sarcoidosis), and hypocitraturia (distal renal tubular acidosis). Obesity is also associated with an increased risk of kidney stones, especially in women with a BMI over 40 [16].

Calcium oxalate stones constitute the majority (60%) of all renal stones, followed by calcium phosphate types (hydroxyapatite 20% and brushite 2%) and struvite stones (7–13%) usually composed of calcium-magnesium-ammonium phosphate. Struvite stones are formed secondary to urease positive bacterial infection and the most common composition of staghorn calculi. If struvite stones do not contain calcium like cystine stones, they become radiolucent and they are missed in radiographs.

Another radiolucent stone is uric acid stone with varying prevalence from 40% in Israel to 10% in the USA [16]. Hyperuricosuria, acidic urine, and low urinary volume are predisposing factors for urate stone. Radiolucent stones can be detected with ultrasound as well as calcium stones.

The main aims of imaging in patients with nephrolithiasis are to assess the size, number, and location of the stone(s), to reveal if there are complications, and to evaluate the contralateral kidney. Ultrasound can be applied to show dilatation of the collecting system, to identify stones, to assess the renal size and renal cortical thickness, and to detect complications. Hydration is very important before the examination, which increases the sensitivity from 24–73% to 85–100%, and increases the specificity from 74 to 83–100% [16, 18].

The composition of the stone does not affect the diagnostic sensitivity and specificity of ultrasound, while the calculus size and position and the body habitus may affect the detection rate along with the experience of the examiner.

The typical appearance of kidney stones is hyperechoic foci with acoustic shadowing (**Figure 3**). Kidney stones need to be at least 4–5 mm to be identified conspicuously on ultrasound [16]. For better visualization, the most appropriate transducer frequency tissue should be considered with a balance of tissue penetration and resolution. The focal zone should be adjusted at the level of stone for maximized shadowing. Furthermore, the detection of kidney stones and the visibility of posterior shadowing are significantly improved by tissue harmonic imaging [19]. Concomitant ultrasound findings in a patient with inflammation due to renal colic are increased echogenicity of renal parenchyma, dilatation of the collecting system, and subcapsular collections (urinomas). The application of color Doppler ultrasound which reveals twinkling artifact posteriorly in 83% of kidney stones improves the detection of small calculi [20].

Several mimickers for kidney stones at ultrasound may result in false-positive diagnosis, including intrarenal gas, renal artery calcification, calcified sloughed papilla, calcified transitional cell tumor, alkaline-encrusted pyelitis, and encrusted ureteral stents.

Nephrocalcinosis is a condition that is caused by hypercalcemia and hypercalciuria due to various diseases. Histologically, tissue calcification can be classified into two groups: calcification in normal and abnormal tissue. Dystrophic calcification arises in abnormal tissues such as vessels, haematoma, tumors, and inflammatory masses and when the solubility of the product of calcium and phosphate is exceeded due to pH changes or a reparative process. This is not considered to be

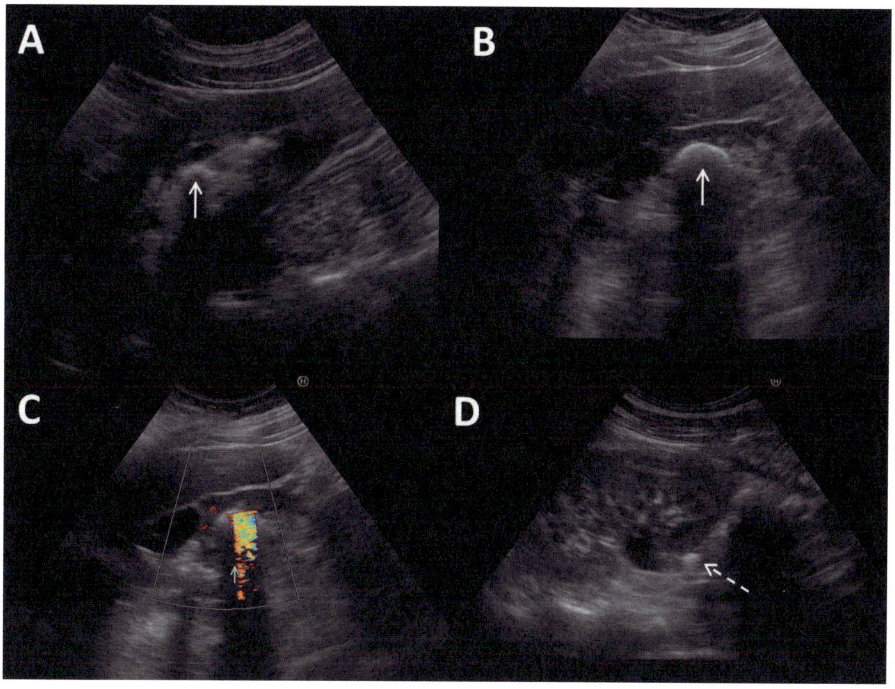

Figure 3.
Examples of kidney stone (arrow) in image (A–C) as a hyperechogenic lesion with acoustic shadowing. In image (D), proximal ureteric stone (dashed arrow) and collecting system dilatation due to obstruction are demonstrated.

nephrocalcinosis. On the other hand, metastatic calcification occurs in normal tissues such as kidneys. It is usually due to abnormal biochemistry, that is, elevated serum calcium. The metabolic imbalance results in metastatic calcification when the solubility of calcium and phosphate or oxalates in extracellular fluid is exceeded.

Metastatic calcification in kidney is further subdivided anatomically into medullary nephrocalcinosis or cortical nephrocalcinosis. Medullary nephrocalcinosis accounts for the 97.6% of nephrocalcinosis and common causes are hyperparathyroidism, renal tubular acidosis, medullary sponge kidney, bone metastases, chronic pyelonephritis, Cushing's syndrome, hyperthyroidism, malignancy, renal papillary necrosis, sarcoidosis, sickle cell disease, hypervitaminosis D, and Wilson's disease. Cortical nephrocalcinosis constitutes the remaining 2.4%, and the common etiologies are acute cortical necrosis, ethylene glycol poisoning, chronic glomerulonephritis, chronic hypercalcemic states, sickle cell disease, and rejected renal transplants [21].

Cortical nephrocalcinosis is seen outlining of the kidney and along the columns of Bertin. It is usually due to severe destructive cortical disease, often observed in patients with end-stage renal failure. Any form of chronic glomerulonephritis may result in cortical nephrocalcinosis. Acute cortical necrosis often related to course of hypovolemic shock and eclampsia may give rise to patchy calcification in the renal parenchyma [16]. Ultrasonographic features of cortical nephrocalcinosis are increased cortical echogenicity representing early cortical calcification. Further progressive calcification may result in hyperechoic rim with extensive shadowing.

Medullary nephrocalcinosis is characterized by diffuse calcium deposition within the renal pyramids. Normally, calcium is removed by lymphatics in renal medulla, and if the amount of calcium exceeds lymphatic capacity, calcium deposits in the fornical tip and margins of the medulla. The typical ultrasound features of early medullary nephrocalcinosis may be nonshadowing echogenic rims surrounding medullary pyramids (**Figure 4**). As the disease progresses, hyperechogenicity fills the entire

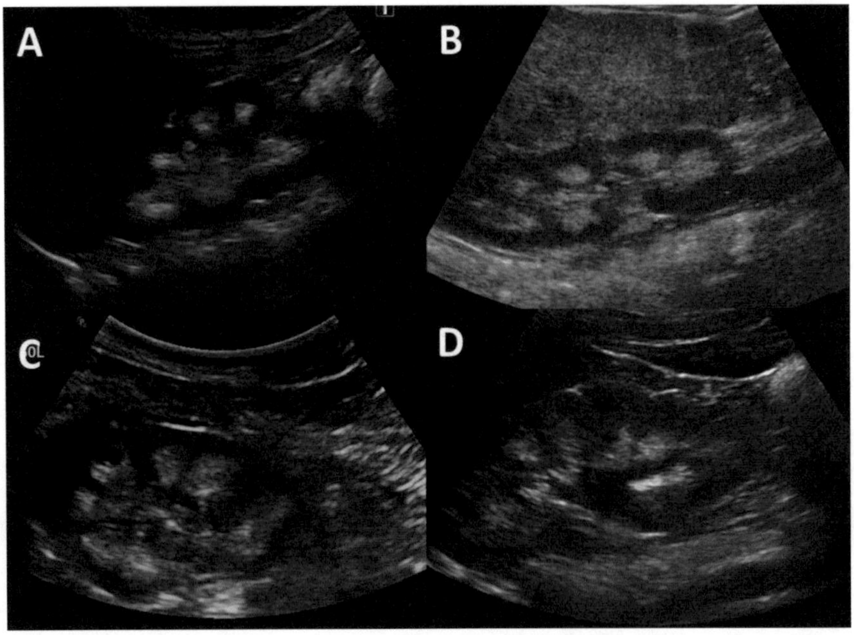

Figure 4.
Four patients with medullary nephrocalcinosis due to different etiology, such as hyperparathyroidism (A), Wilson's disease (B), and medullary sponge kidney (C and D). In all patients, the calyceal system is seen hyperechogenic.

pyramids. However, increased medullary echogenicity may also be seen in medullary sponge kidney; even it may be a physiologic transient finding in neonates [22]. In a similar way to cortical nephrocalcinosis, further calcium deposition induces acoustic shadowing at ultrasound in medullary nephrocalcinosis. These firm calcifications may perforate the caliceal wall and compose a nidus for further stone formation.

6. Cystic disease of kidney

Renal cystic disease is an entity that includes an enormous range of disorders including developmental (simple and complex cysts, localized cystic diseases, extraparenchymal sinus cysts, medullary sponge kidney, and multicystic dysplastic kidney), acquired (acquired cystic kidney disease), and hereditary (autosomal dominant polycystic kidney disease, autosomal recessive polycystic kidney disease, tuberous sclerosis complex, and von Hippel– Lindau disease) origin. Ultrasound is the primary and the most commonly used imaging modality for cystic renal disease but insufficient for the exact diagnosis in most of the cases. Key imaging features are the location, distribution, size, and composition of renal cysts as well as other coexisting noncystic renal lesions for the diagnosis [23].

Simple renal cysts are benign, fluid filled homogenous, and asymptomatic lesions, most of which are incidentally discovered on ultrasound. Prevalence of simple cysts increases with age in up to 27% of patients greater than 50 years of age [24]. They can be single or multiple, unilateral or bilateral, and commonly located in the renal cortex. Simple cysts are typically anechoic, round, or ovoid, with acoustic enhancement and no prominent wall thickness (**Figure 5**). If all these features are met with ultrasound, further evaluation or follow-up of the cyst is not required. All other sonographic findings, such as internal echo, septum, wall thickening, calcification, or acoustic shadowing, lead to the diagnosis of complex cyst.

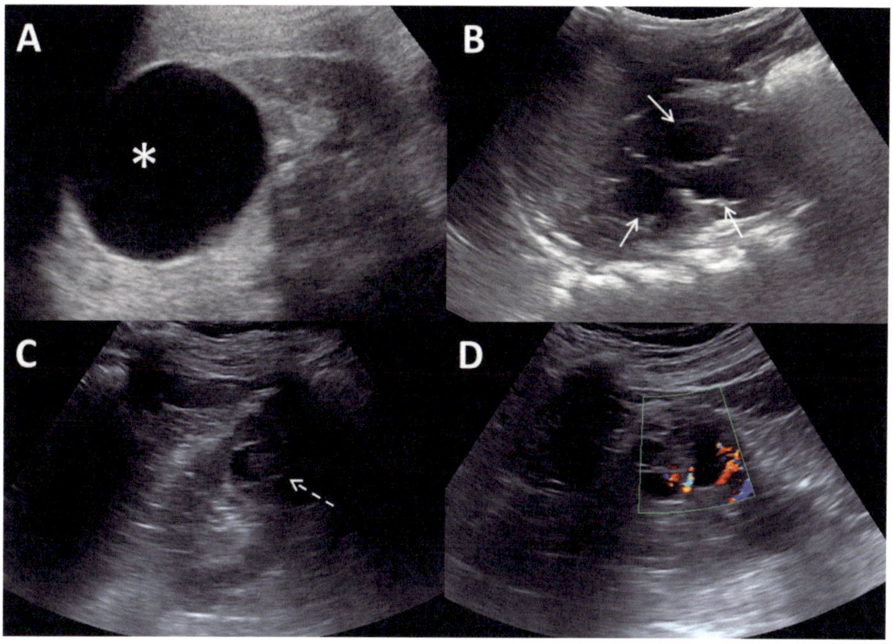

Figure 5.
Simple cyst of the kidney (asterix) should be purely anechoic with no septations and solid component (A). Also increased trough transmission can be seen posteriorly. Hydronephrosis (B) is seen as a multiple cystic structure (arrows) which is actually dilated calyx. In image (C), cystic lesion with multiple irregular septations is demonstrated (dashed arrow). On color Doppler ultrasound (D), vascularity in the septations is shown. Histopathologic evaluation confirmed the diagnosis of this cystic lesion as a clear cell type renal cell carcinoma.

Internal echoes within a cyst are generally due to hemorrhage or infection as in septations. Calcification can be seen in cyst wall or septa and may be fine and linear or amorphous and thick according to the shape. Thin wall or septal calcification suggests a complicated cyst rather than malignancy, while thick, irregular, amorphous calcification, perceptible, thickened walls, or mural nodularity should raise suspicion for malignancy, and further contrast enhanced imaging should be done (**Figure 5C,D**). Layering milk of calcium is seen as an echogenic focus with ring-down arifact in septa or cyst wall suggest that the cyst has a benign nature [25].

The most widely used classification system for complex renal cysts was introduced in 1991 by Bosniak [26], who grouped renal cysts into five categories based on imaging appearance in an attempt to predict the risk of malignancy and determine the outcome and management of complex cysts and cystic neoplasm (**Table 1**).

Extraparenchymal cysts are commonly seen in renal sinus and subdivided into parapelvic cyst and peripelvic cyst. Parapelvic cysts originate from the renal parenchyma and extend into the renal sinus, while peripelvic cysts arise directly in the renal sinus presumably due to lymphatic obstruction. Although these cysts differ in their origin, they are indistinguishable sonographically and benign nature, without a need for further imaging and follow up. However, these cysts may mimic hydronephrosis. Shape and extension of the cyst and concomitant caliceal dilatation of hydronephrosis are useful findings for differentiation [23].

Medullary cystic disease and juvenile nephronophthisis have similar imaging findings that are both composed of small multiple cysts at the corticomedullary junction and medulla. Juvenile nephronophthisis is an autosomal recessive condition usually present in childhood and generally progresses to end stage renal disease. On the other hand, medullary cystic disease is an autosomal dominant disorder present in the third or fourth decade of life with similar renal symptoms.

Autosomal dominant polycystic kidney disease (ADPKD) is the most common inherited renal disorder that is characterized by the progressive development of multiple asymmetrical and different sized cysts and marked renal enlargement [28]. ADPKD accounts for 10–15% of patients receiving dialysis and is the fourth leading cause of end stage renal disease in the world [23, 25]. Ultrasound is commonly used as a screening tool for the children of affected individuals (**Figure 6A**). According to Pei et al. [29], when evaluating patients with a positive family history of ADPKD, the number of renal cysts required for diagnosis is at least three (unilateral or bilateral) in subjects between 15 and 39 years old, at least two in each kidney in subjects between 40 and 59 years old, and at least four in each kidney in subjects more than 60 years old. Most of the cysts are simple cysts with varying size, which may be complicated by hemorrhage or infection and have thick walls, internal echoes, and/or fluid debris levels. Calcification in the cyst wall or stones may be seen as echogenic foci with acoustic shadowing. Most common associated extrarenal cysts of ADPKD are seen in liver, followed by pancreas, spleen, epididymis, seminal vesicle, uterus, ovary and thyroid [23]. Cerebral berry aneurysms, abdominal aortic aneurysm, cardiac valve diseases, and colonic diverticula may also accompany [25].

Autosomal recessive polycystic kidney disease (ARPKD) is characterized by renal tubular ectasia (manifesting as multiple bilateral renal cysts) and hepatic ductal plate malformation (leading to hepatic fibrosis and Caroli's disease) [23]. It is divided into four types depending on the age of onset: antenatal, neonatal, infantile, and juvenile forms. In the earlier age group, the more severe renal findings and the less pronounced hepatic involvement are encountered [30]. Ultrasound features of renal-dominant ARPKD include a lack of corticomedullary differentiation and massively enlarged, echogenic kidneys (**Figure 6B**). The increased echogenicity is due to the unresolved 1–2 mm cystic dilatation of the collecting tubules, which increases the number of acoustic interfaces. In neonates, small cysts may be revealed more clearly with high frequency linear-arrayed transducers.

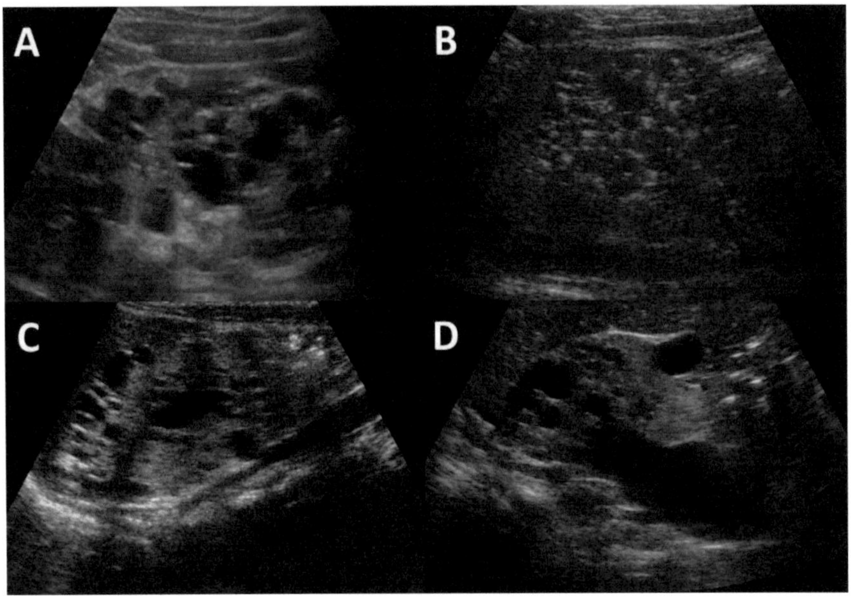

Figure 6.
Ultrasound images of different renal cystic diseases, autosomal dominant polycystic kidney disease (A), autosomal recessive polycystic kidney disease (B), acquired cysts after chronic dialysis with end stage renal disease (C), and cystic renal dysplasia of newborn (D).

Localized cystic disease is a rare, benign condition that may mimic ADPKD. It is characterized by a cluster of simple cysts localized in either a portion of kidney (segmental cystic disease of the kidney) or an entire kidney (unilateral cystic disease of the kidney) [31]. On ultrasound, it appears as a conglomerate mass of multiple cysts of varying size separated by normal or atrophic kidney parenchyma. Lack of cysts in the contralateral kidney and other organs differentiates the disease from ADPKD [25].

Acquired cystic kidney disease (ACKD) is a progressive disorder, which occurs in the native kidneys of patients with end stage renal disease undergoing either chronic hemodialysis or peritoneal dialysis (**Figure 6C**). The prevalence of ACKD depends on the duration of dialysis and accounts for 40–60% of patients by 5 years and over 90% by 10 years of dialysis. Although the affected kidneys are usually atrophic at the time of cyst development, they may have an enlarged appearance due to the formation of extensive renal cysts and thus resemble ADPKD in some cases [32]. Three to five cysts in each kidney at ultrasound and increase in number in follow-up in a patient with chronic dialysis are diagnostics for ACKD [25].

Multicystic dysplastic kidney (MCDK) is a nonhereditary, developmental disorder characterized by multiple renal cysts replacing functional kidney parenchyma in the affected entire or segmented kidney which is smaller and has a distorted appearance. It is the most common cystic disease in pediatric population with an incidence of 1:4000. The exact etiology is unclear but proposed underlying causes are genetic disturbances, teratogens, in utero infections, and more commonly urinary tract outflow obstruction [33]. Ipsilateral renal anomalies, such as vesicoureteral reflux, or contralateral renal anomalies such as ureteropelvic junction obstruction are usually associated with MCDK. Typical sonographic findings include multiple cysts without communication, absence of normal parenchyma, and renal sinus among the cysts. Focal hyperechoic areas representing primitive mesenchyma or tiny cysts can be seen between the cysts [25]. Since many of the MDCKs involute over time, follow-up with ultrasound is recommended and nephrectomy should be reserved for the cases with hypertension, malignant transformation, or exceptionally large cystic kidneys [34].

Cystic renal dysplasia is the consequence of a developmental anomaly composed of abnormal structural organization and development of metanephric elements (**Figure 6D**). Both kidneys are affected and may have multiple cysts. It is often associated with urinary tract obstruction and may be seen with posterior urethral valve, prune belly syndrome, and ureteropelvic junction obstruction. This suggests that obstruction and urinary retention may cause anomalous kidney development [35].

Multilocular cystic nephroma (MLCN) is a rare benign disorder, composed of multiple noncommunicating cysts contained within a well-defined capsule and occasionally affects both kidneys. It has a trimodal age distribution that is seen in male patients less than 4 years of age and in female patients aged 4–20 or 40–60 years. MLCN is generally asymptomatic or may present with abdominal pain, hematuria, and hypertension. If the cysts of MLCN are tiny, a more solid-appearing echogenic mass will be present that precludes to differentiate MLCN from cystic RCC with ultrasound [25].

Chronic lithium nephropathy (CLN) is caused by long-term treatment with lithium salts that result in chronic tubulointerstitial nephropathy. In up to 62% of cases with CLN, typical findings of multiple small cysts (<2 mm) localized in both the cortex and the medulla uniformly and symmetrically distributed are observed [36]. Due to small size, cysts may not be recognized with ultrasound in some patients and magnetic resonance imaging is required for delineation.

7. Solid kidney lesions

Angiomyolipoma (AML) is the most frequent mesenchymal benign neoplasms of the kidney with a prevalence of 0.3–3% and with a female preponderance [37]. It is composed of varying amounts of adipose tissue, smooth muscle cells, and blood vessels [25]. It is frequently associated with an autosomal dominant phakomatosis syndrome, and with lymphangioleiomyomatosis, a progressive disease which usually affects the lungs of young women and which is also related to tuberous sclerosis. In up to 80% children with tuberous sclerosis, AMLs are usually seen as bilateral, small, and multifocal. However, in sporadic patients, AMLs are typically unilateral and discovered in middle-aged women.

Small AMLs typically appear as homogenous hyperechoic lesion, sharply marginated with detectable shadowing (**Figure 7**). Since larger AMLs may be more heterogeneous, it may be difficult to differentiate them from RCC and retroperitoneal liposarcoma. Magnetic resonance imaging should be indicated for these lesions. AMLs may rarely behave locally aggressive, with infiltration to the adjacent lymph nodes or within the inferior vena cava. Small, asymptomatic AMLs may be followed but if they are larger than 3–4 cm, they may be complicated by hemorrhage, which can be spontaneous or associated with relatively minor or incidental trauma. Bleeding may occur either within the tumor, or in the adjacent renal parenchyma, subcapsular, or retroperitoneal area. Complicated AMLs are treated surgically or by selective embolization [38].

Due to the lack of lymphoid tissue in the normal kidney, lymphomatous involvement of the kidney occurs from either hematogenous dissemination or from infiltration of retroperitoneal disease [25]. The kidneys are the 6th most affected abdominal organ after spleen, liver, gastrointestinal tract, pancreas, and abdominal wall [39]. Renal involvement is usually bilateral and found in one third of lymphoma patients at autopsy series [25]. Five different ultrasound appearances are recognized for renal lymphoma, depending partially on the growth pattern of the tumor: (1) single mass, (2) multiple masses, (3) infiltrative disease, (4) perirenal disease, and (5) invasion from retroperitoneal disease [40]. Focal masses appear as hypoechoic or anechoic homogenous lesions. If they are anechoic, they can be differentiated from cysts with the absence of increased through-transmission behind the lesion [25]. Diffuse infiltration may usually enlarge the kidney and decrease echogenicity despite disruption of renal architecture. Isolated perirenal involvement is very rare (<10% of cases of perirenal lymphoma) and appears as a soft tissue mass involving the perirenal space partially or completely and compresses but does not infiltrate the kidney [40]. Perirenal disease is frequently a part of retroperitoneal extension. Perirenal or retroperitoneal tumor may be confused with hematoma or extramedullary hematopoiesis. The lack of renal venous invasion, despite extensive retroperitoneal and renal sinus invasion, may help in differentiating renal lymphoma from renal cell carcinoma (RCC). Contrast-enhanced CT and MRI are superior to ultrasound for diagnosis of renal lymphoma (higher sensitivity and specificity) and in evaluating the extent of disease [40].

Leukemia involves the kidney either diffusely or with focal masses. Leukemic infiltration of the kidney has been reported in 65% of patients at autopsy series [25]. Although the typical ultrasound appearance of renal leukemia is bilateral kidney enlargement, in 15% of the leukemia patients, the kidney may enlarge without leukemic infiltration [25]. Renal leukemia may also be manifested as single or multiple focal masses or a coarsened parenchymal echo pattern with a distorted central sinus echo complex. These patients are more prone to renal, subcapsular, perirenal, or retroperitoneal bleeding.

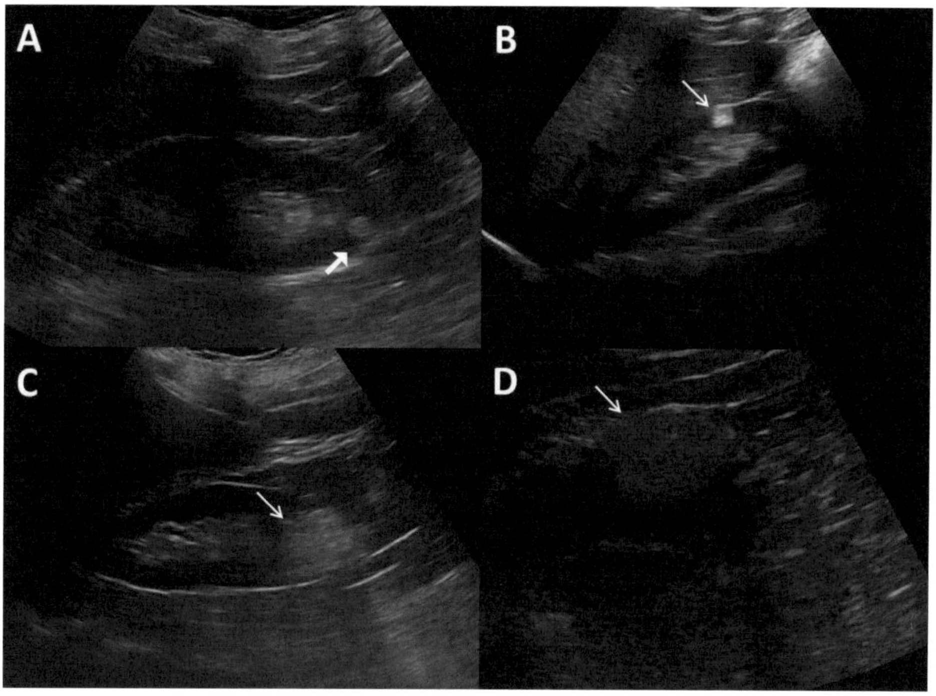

Figure 7.
Different patients with angiomyolipoma (arrows) with different sizes (A, B, C, D). Although appearances of the lesions are different, they are typically hyperechogenic.

Renal cell carcinoma (RCC) is the most common primary kidney malignancy in adults and constitutes 86% of all primary malignant renal tumors and 3% of all adult malignancies [25]. RCC most often occurs in patients aged 50–70 years with 2:1 male predominance [41]. Most of the RCCs appear solid on ultrasound without any specific echogenicity. Smaller RCCs are more hyperechoic and can be misdiagnosed as AML at ultrasound. Several distinguishing characteristics are hypoechoic rim or cystic spaces more common in RCCs, while weak posterior acoustic shadowing can be seen more often in AMLs [25].

The most common subtype of RCC is clear cell (70–75%), followed by papillary (15%), chromophobe (5%), and oncocytic (2–3%) subtypes [25]. The last three have much better prognosis than clear cell RCC. Although ultrasound is much less accurate than CT or MRI for characterization of tumor content, lack of cystic necrotic areas and the presence of calcification, which are more common in papillary and chromophobe subtypes, appear to be associated with a better prognosis. Ultrasound may also demonstrate additional findings related to RCCs, including hydronephrosis; vascular encasement with diminished Doppler flow to the area of involvement or deterioration of the normal central sinus echo complex may be seen [41].

Cystic RCCs account for 5–7% of all RCCs. Four subtypes have been described for cystic RCCs at ultrasound: (1) unilocular, (2) multilocular, (3) necrotic (cystic necrosis), and (4) tumors emerging in a simple cyst. Since the unilocular and multilocular subtypes behave less aggressive, recognition of subtypes may have clinical importance [25]. The typical sonographic features of a unilocular RCC are a debris-filled mass with thick, irregular capsule that may have calcifications. Multilocular RCC may manifest as a cystic mass with internal septations which are thick (>2 mm) and nodular and may contain calcification. Necrotic RCCs have varying appearance depending on the degree of tumor necrosis. RCCs originating in a simple cyst are very rare and usually seen in Von Hippel Lindau disease patients. A solid mural nodule can be seen at the base of a simple cyst at ultrasound.

Transitional cell carcinoma (TCC) of the renal pelvis is the second most common primary kidney tumor with a prevalence of 7%, but it is 50 times less common than bladder TCCs. Renal TCCs are typically seen in elderly men who are admitted with gross or microscopic hematuria in 75% and flank pain in 25%. The variable appearance of renal sinus beclouds the evaluation of renal pelvis TCCs. Patients at increased risk for development of TCC (such as patients with Balkan nephritis, vesicoureteral reflux, analgesic abuse, heavy smoking habit, exposure to carcinogens, or cyclophosphamide therapy) may require close follow-up. Papillary TCCs appear as solid, central, hypoechoic masses in renal with or without associated proximal calyceal dilatation. The differential diagnosis of these masses includes fibrin clots, sloughed papillae, and mycetoma [25].

Kidney metastases are usually seen on imaging for staging without any symptoms and have an incidence of 2–20% at autopsy series. Renal involvement is generally due to hematogenous spread. The most common primary tumor that metastasizes to kidney is lung carcinoma followed by breast carcinoma and RCC of the contralateral kidney [25]. Colon adenocarcinoma usually has solitary metastasis as a solid lesion on ultrasound which is indistinguishable from RCC [25]. Involvement of perirenal and retroperitoneal space is particularly seen in malignant melanoma and lung cancer metastasis [25]. Infiltrating metastases with subtle margins may be misdiagnosed with ultrasound and contrast enhanced imaging is required for further delineation.

8. Infections

Acute pyelonephritis is defined as an inflammation of the kidney and renal pelvis and has typical symptoms consisting of an abrupt onset of chills, high-grade fever (>38.5°C), and unilateral or bilateral flank pain with costovertebral tenderness. Middle aged females are most commonly affected and *Escherichia coli* is by far the most common pathogen accounting for 80% of community-acquired and 50% of hospital-acquired infections most frequently due to ascending urinary tract infections [42]. In children, recurrent pyelonephritis commonly occurs as a result of vesicoureteral reflux.

The vast majority of acute pyelonephritis patients have normal findings on ultrasound. However, the following findings of pyelonephritis may be identified: kidney enlargement, abnormal echogenicity, loss of corticomedullary differentiation, ill-defined hyperechoic mass (es) (in focal pyelonephritis), compression of the renal sinus, and gas within kidney parenchyma (emphysematous pyelonephritis) (**Figure 8**). Untreated acute pyelonephritis may complicate with necrosis and abscess formation. Acute abscesses usually appear as a hypoechoic mass with increased through transmission posteriorly and indistinct margins. Over time, the abscess wall will be thickened and fluid levels will be developed within the abscess cavity [42]. Emphysematous pyelonephritis (EPN) is a rare, life-threatening infection seen in diabetic patients characterized by gas formation in the renal parenchyma. Dirty shadowing is revealed on ultrasound in EPN and contrast enhanced CT should be preferred for imaging to determine the location and extent of renal and perinephric gas [25].

Fungal infections of the kidney usually affect patients with diabetes mellitus, chronic indwelling catheters, malignancy, chronic antibiotic or steroid therapy, transplantation, and IV drug abusers [43]. *Candida albicans* is the most common fungal agent involved in genitourinary infections. Fungal infections usually manifest as unilateral small parenchymal abscesses which are tiny, hypoechoic, cortical

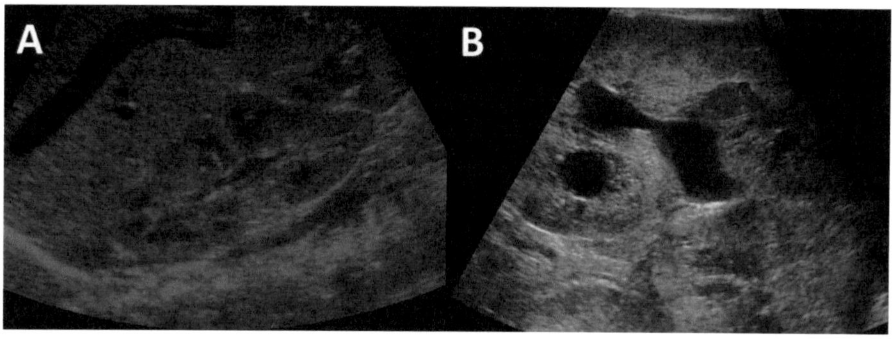

Figure 8.
Two patients with acute pyelonephritis (A and B). Although the majority of the acute pyelonephritis has normal ultrasound appearance, in severe form of the disease, kidney enlargement and increased echogenicity of the kidney can be seen. In image (B), collecting duct dilatation is also seen which might be due to obstructive stone in the ureter.

lesions that may calcify over time [25]. Invasion of the collecting system results in fungus balls which are seen as hyperechoic soft tissue masses without posterior acoustic shadowing within the collecting system [43]. Fungus balls are motile and cause obstruction that may be associated with varying degrees of hydronephrosis on ultrasound.

9. Trauma

Renal injury occurs in 8–10% of patients suffering from blunt or penetrating trauma [44]. Blunt injury is far more common than penetrating injury accounting for 66–90% of cases and the majority of blunt trauma patients have relatively minor injuries which heal without any treatment. While blunt injuries are most often caused by motor vehicle accidents, falls, and direct impact from assault or sports competition, penetrating injuries are usually the result of gunshot or stab wounds. Patients with renal lesions (such as cysts, tumor, or hydronephrosis) are more prone to severe injury. The broadly accepted renal injury grading system constituted by the American Association for the Surgery of Trauma (AAST) is shown in **Table 1** [27].

Most patients with grade I and II injury are managed conservatively, while grades IV and V often require surgical treatment [27]. Contrast enhanced computed

AAST injury grading	Description
Grade I	Renal contusion or subcapsular hematoma with intact capsule
Grade II	Superficial cortex laceration (≤1 cm) that does not extend to deep medulla or the collecting system or nonexpanding hematoma
Grade III	Deep laceration(s) (>1 cm) with or without urine Extravasation
Grade IV	Laceration(s) extending into the collecting system with contained urine leak
Grade V	Shattered kidney, renal vascular pedicle injury, or devitalized kidney

Table 1.
Renal injury grading scale of the American Association for the Surgery of Trauma [27].

tomography is the premier imaging modality for the evaluation of renal trauma. Technical limitations usually hinder an adequate examination with ultrasound in trauma patients. However, ultrasound may be used in the follow-up of patients with known kidney trauma [25]. Renal hematomas may be revealed as hypoechoic, hyperechoic, or heterogeneous depending on the stage of blood products. Lacerations are seen as linear hypoechoic defects that may extend through the kidney if a fracture is present and perinephric collections are associated with them. Subcapsular hemorrhage may appear as a perinephric heterogeneous fluid collection that flattens the underlying renal border. A shattered kidney in grade V trauma consists of multiple fragments of disorganized tissue with associated hemorrhage without normal renal architecture and urine collection in the renal bed.

10. Conclusion

Typical US features of the normal kidney and normal anatomic variants are very important to prevent over diagnosis and to recognize pathologic lesions. Moreover, typical US findings of benign lesions are extremely important to prevent unnecessary additional imaging and interventions. Although US is the first-line imaging and the second-line cross-sectional imaging modalities (CT and MRI) are performed in malignant disorders, radiologists and clinicians should be familiar with typical US appearances to narrow down differential diagnosis, to guide for most appropriate second-line imaging and for comprehensive follow-up.

Acknowledgements

The images are obtained from the archives of Istanbul Medeniyet University and Bingol State Hospital radiology archives.

Conflict of interest

The author declares no conflict of interest about this chapter.

Author details

Ercan Ayaz
Department of Radiology, Hacettepe University School of Medicine, Ankara, Turkey

*Address all correspondence to: ercan.ayaz1@gmail.com

References

[1] Zweyer M. Embryology of the kidney. In: Quaia E, editor. Radiological Imaging of the Kidney. Medical Radiology. Berlin, Heidelberg: Springer; 2010. pp. 3-16

[2] Moore KL, Dalley AF, Agur AMR. Clinically Oriented Anatomy. 6th ed. Philedelphia: Wolters Kluwer/Lippincott Williams & Wilkins; 2010

[3] Quaia E, Martingano P, Cavallaro M, Zappetti R. Normal radiological anatomy and anatomical variants of the kidney. In: Quaia E, editor. Radiological Imaging of the Kidney. Medical Radiology. Berlin, Heidelberg: Springer; 2014. pp. 17-74

[4] Emamian SA, Nielsen MB, Pedersen JF, Ytte L. Kidney dimensions at sonography: Correlation with age, sex, and habitus in 665 adult volunteers. American Journal of Roentgenology. 1993;**160**:83-86

[5] Netter FH. Anatomy, structure, and embryology. In: Shapter RK, Yonkman FF, editors. The CIBA Collection of Medical Illustrations, Vol. 6. Kidneys, Ureters, and Urinary Bladder. Summit, NJ, USA: CIBA Pharmaceutical; 1973. pp. 2-35

[6] Friedenberg RM, Dunbar JS. Excretory urography. In: Pollack HM, editor. Clinical Urography. Philadelphia: Saunders; 1990. pp. 101-243

[7] Platt JF, Rubin JM, Bowerman RA, Marn CS. The inability to detect kidney disease on the basis of echogenicity. American Journal of Roentgenology. 1988;**151**:317-319

[8] Kasap B, Soylu A, Türkmen M, et al. Relationship of increased renal cortical echogenicity with clinical and laboratory findings in pediatric renal disease. Journal of Clinical Ultrasound. 2006;**34**:339-342

[9] Yeh HC, Halton KP, Shapiro RS, et al. Junctional parenchyma: Revised definition of hypertrophic column of Bertin. Radiology. 1992;**185**:725-732

[10] Leekam RN, Matzinger MA, Brunelle M, et al. The sonography of renal columnar hypertrophy. Journal of Clinical Ultrasound. 1983;**11**:491-494

[11] Quaia E. Ultrasound of the kidney. In: Quaia E, editor. Radiological Imaging of the Kidney. Medical Radiology. Berlin, Heidelberg: Springer; 2014. pp. 83-121

[12] Friedland GW, Devries PA, Nino-Murcia M, et al. Congenital anomalies of the urinary tract. In: Pollack HM, editor. Clinical Urography: An Atlas and Textbook of Urologic Imaging. Philadelphia, USA: Saunders; 1990. pp. 559-787

[13] Talner LB. Specific causes of obstruction. In: Pollack HM, editor. Clinical Urography: An Atlas and Textbook of Urological Imaging. Philadelphia: Saunders; 1990. pp. 1629-1751

[14] Menon M, Resnick MI. Urinary lithiasis: Etiology, diagnosis, and medical management. In: Walsh PC, Retik AB, Darracott VE Jr, editors. Campbell's Urology. Philadelphia, USA: WB Saunders; 2002. pp. 3229-3305

[15] Sandhu C, Anson KM, Patel U. Urinary tract stones–Part I: Role of radiological imaging in diagnosis and treatment planning. Clinical Radiology. 2003;**58**:415-421

[16] Phillips S, Tudor GR. Nephrocalcinosis and nephrolithiasis. In: Quaia E, editor. Radiological Imaging of the Kidney. Medical Radiology. Berlin, Heidelberg: Springer; 2014. pp. 391-410

[17] Freeman SJ, Sells S. Investigation of loin pain. Imaging. 2008;**20**:38-56

[18] Fowler KA, Locken JA, Duchesne JH, et al. US for detecting renal calculi with nonenhanced CT as a reference standard. Radiology. 2002;**222**:109-113

[19] Ozdemir H, Demir MK, Temizöz O, et al. Phase inversion harmonic imaging improves assessment of renal calculi: A comparison with fundamental gray-scale sonography. Journal of Clinical Ultrasound. 2008;**36**:16-19

[20] Lee JY, Kim SH, Cho JY, Han D. Color and power Doppler twinkling artifacts from urinary stones: Clinical observations and phantom studies. American Journal of Roentgenology. 2001;**176**:1441-1445

[21] Banner M. Nephrocalcinosis. In: Pollack HM, editor. Clinical Urography: An Atlas and Textbook of Urological Imaging. Philadelphia, USA: Saunders; 1990. pp. 1768-1775

[22] Khoory BJ, Andreis IA, Vino L, Fanos V. Transient hyperechogenicity of the renal medullary pyramids: Incidence in the healthy term newborn. American Journal of Perinatology. 1999;**16**:463-468

[23] Bae KT, Furlan A, Mileto A. Renal cystic disease. In: Quaia E, editor. Radiological Imaging of the Kidney. Medical Radiology. Berlin, Heidelberg: Springer; 2014. pp. 305-334

[24] Tada S, Yamagishi J, Kobayashi H, et al. The incidence of simple renal cyst by computed tomography. Clinical Radiology. 1983;**34**:437-439

[25] Tublin M, Thurston W, Wilson SR. The kidney and urinary tract. In: Rumack CM, Wilson SR, Charboneu JW, Levine D, editors. Diagnostic Ultrasound. 4th ed. Philadelphia, PA, USA: Elsevier Mosby; 2011. pp. 317-391

[26] Bosniak MA. The small (≤3.0 cm) renal parenchymal tumor: Detection, diagnosis, and controversies. Radiology. 1991;**179**:307-317

[27] Kozar RA, Crandall M, Shanmuganathan K, Zarzaur BL, Coburn M, Cribari C, et al. Organ injury scaling 2018 update: Spleen, liver, and kidney. The Journal of Trauma and Acute Care Surgery. 2018;**85**:1119-1122

[28] Harris PC, Bae KT, Rossetti S, et al. Cyst number but not the rate of cystic growth is associated with the mutated gene in autosomal dominant polycystic kidney disease. Journal of the American Society of Nephrology. 2006;**17**:3013-3019

[29] Pei Y, Obaji J, Dupuis A, et al. Unified criteria for ultrasonographic diagnosis of ADPKD. Journal of the American Society of Nephrology. 2009;**20**:205-212

[30] Turkbey B, Ocak I, Daryanani K, et al. Autosomal recessive polycystic kidney disease and congenital hepatic fibrosis (ARPKD/CHF). Pediatric Radiology. 2009;**39**:100-111

[31] Slywotzky CM, Bosniak MA. Localized cystic disease of the kidney. American Journal of Roentgenology. 2001;**176**:843-849

[32] Bakir AA, Hasnain M, Young S, et al. Dialysis-associated renal cystic disease resembling autosomal dominant polycystic kidney disease: A report of two cases. American Journal of Nephrology. 1999;**19**:519-522

[33] Hains DS, Bates CM, Ingraham S, et al. Management and etiology of the unilateral multicystic dysplastic kidney: A review. Pediatric Nephrology. 2009;**24**:233-241

[34] Vester U, Kranz B, Hoyer PF. The diagnostic value of ultrasound in cystic kidney diseases. Pediatric Nephrology. 2010;**25**:231-240

[35] Shibata S, Nagata M. Pathogenesis of human renal dysplasia: An alternative scenario to the major theories. Pediatrics International. 2003;**45**:605-609

[36] Roque A, Heredia V, Ramalho M, et al. MR findings of lithium related kidney disease: Preliminary observations in four patients. Abdominal Imaging. 2012;**37**:140-146

[37] Quaia E. Benign solid renal tumors. In: Quaia E, editor. Radiological Imaging of the Kidney. Medical Radiology. Berlin, Heidelberg: Springer; 2014. pp. 501-535

[38] Silverman SG, Israel GM, Herts BR, et al. Management of the incidental renal mass. Radiology. 2008;**249**:16-31

[39] Lee WK, Lau EW, Duddalwar VA, et al. Abdominal manifestations of extranodal lymphoma: Spectrum of imaging findings. American Journal of Roentgenology. 2008;**191**:198-206

[40] Rappaport A, Oyen RH. Renal lymphoma and renal sarcoma. In: Quaia E, editor. Radiological Imaging of the Kidney. Medical Radiology. Berlin, Heidelberg: Springer; 2014. pp. 631-643

[41] Hayashi D, Guermazi A, Holalkere NS. Imaging in renal cell carcinoma. In: Quaia E, editor. Radiological Imaging of the Kidney. Medical Radiology. Berlin, Heidelberg: Springer; 2014. pp. 537-570

[42] Blandino A, Mazziotti S, Minutoli F, Ascenti G, Gaeta M. Acute renal infections. In: Quaia E, editor. Radiological Imaging of the Kidney. Medical Radiology. Berlin, Heidelberg: Springer; 2014. pp. 411-436

[43] Quaia E, Giarraputo L, Martingano P, Cavallaro M. Chronic renal infections and renal fungal infections. In: Quaia E, editor. Radiological Imaging of the Kidney. Medical Radiology. Berlin, Heidelberg: Springer; 2014. pp. 437-467

[44] Mirvis SE. Imaging of renal trauma. In: Quaia E, editor. Radiological Imaging of the Kidney. Medical Radiology. Berlin, Heidelberg: Springer; 2014. pp. 483-498

[45] Behrman RE, Kliegman RM, Arvin AM. Nelson Textbook of Pediatrics. 15th ed. Philadelphia: WB Saunders; 1996

Section 5

Doppler Ultrasound of the Kidneys

Chapter 5

Ultrasound of the Kidneys: Application of Doppler and Elastography

Moawia Gameraddin

Abstract

Doppler ultrasound of the kidneys is essential in the assessment and diagnosis of kidney diseases. There are several diseases involving the kidneys. Some are functional, diffuse and systematic. Using Doppler imaging provides an assessment of vascular changes which is easily evaluated. Doppler investigation is widely used for assessment of the perfusion of renal arteries. The Doppler indexes; resistive index, pulsatility index, peak systolic are utilized for evaluating the blood flow of the renal arteries. Doppler analysis provides useful diagnostic data that can predict early damage of the kidney tissue. In recent years, ultrasound elastography showed advanced development. It is a new promising technique that is used for assessing the renal tissue characterization. Elastography is an effective imaging for assessing kidney diseases. In the future, clinicians can use elastography instead of biopsy. In this chapter, we highlighted the applications of Doppler ultrasound and elastography in evaluation of various kidney diseases.

Keywords: Doppler, renal elastography, kidney disease, renal artery

1. Introduction

Doppler ultrasound is widely used in medical imaging. It is an application of diagnostic ultrasound utilized for assessing the blood flow speed and direction. These measurements depend on the Doppler effect is used to measure changes in the frequency of the echoes reflected from moving blood cells. In many cases, Doppler ultrasound replaces X-ray angiography. The most important advantage of Doppler ultrasound over other imaging methods that it provides a real-time assessment of blood flow.

The Doppler renal resistive index (RRI) is the most common Doppler parameter that is used to assess a variety of renal diseases such as assessment of rejection of transplanted kidney, detection of renal artery stenosis in hypertensive patients and evaluation of chronic kidney disease (CKD).

Ultrasound elastography is an advanced imaging method which is sensitive to tissue stiffness. In recent years, elastography has been further developed to enable quantitative assessments of tissue stiffness. Elastography is capable to assess changed elasticity of soft tissues resulting from specific pathological processes. It can differentiate between malignant and benign renal masses which may replace the need of biopsy. The combination of Doppler and elastography provide rich diagnostic data about the pathological processes with kidney tissue which is essential for management and treatment.

 IntechOpen

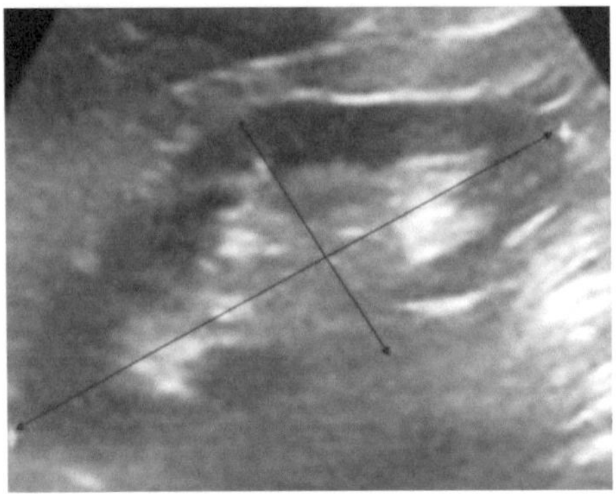

Figure 1.
The length and width of the kidney.

1.1 Ultrasound examination technique

The kidneys are examined with ultrasound in longitudinal and transverse scans planes using 3.5 and 5 MHz transducers. The organ is examined in supine position combined with the lateral decubitus. Then various planes are performed to demonstrate the entire kidney. Preferably, longitudinal and transverse planes are taken to determine the length and size of the kidney, as shown in **Figure 1**.

In the adult patient, a curved array transducer with of 2.5–3.5 MHz is used, while high-frequency 5–7 MHz is used in the pediatric patients.

Artifacts of the lowest ribs and gastric gases may obscure the upper poles of the kidneys. However, the whole kidney can be investigated during either normal respiration or breath hold, since the kidney will follow the diaphragm movement and change position accordingly [1].

2. The Doppler ultrasound: a general review

Doppler ultrasound has been extensively utilized in assessing reno-vascular diseases since it is a safe, non-invasive, available and cheap. These measurements depend on the Doppler effect is used to measure changes in the frequency of the echoes reflected from moving blood cells. In many cases, Doppler ultrasound replaces X-ray angiography. The most important advantage of Doppler ultrasound over other imaging methods that it provides a real-time assessment of blood flow.

2.1 Types of Doppler ultrasound imaging

All kinds of Doppler sonography are widely used in medical imaging. The advantages of these types are high accuracy in measurements, non-invasive nature, accessibility, and no harmful biological effects. Today, there are three types:

a. Color Doppler

b. Power Doppler

c. Pulse wave Doppler

The color Doppler (CD) converts Doppler shifts to an array of colors and form a picture of blood vessels to display the speed and direction of blood flow through the vessels. The Doppler shift is the difference between the incident frequency and reflected frequency. Positive Doppler shift occurs when the reflector is moving away from the probe, and a negative shift occurs when the reflector moving toward the source of ultrasound. Thus, the Doppler shift is directly proportional to the velocity of the blood flow.

$$FD = \frac{2F0v\ cos\ 0}{C} \tag{1}$$

where F_0: is the transmitted ultrasound frequency; V: is the reflector velocity; C: is the speed of sound; Cos 0: is the cosine of the angle between the transmitted beam and the reflector path.

2.1.1 Factors influencing color flow image

1. Power: transmitted power into tissue*

2. Gain: affect sensitivity to flow signals

3. Frequency: affect sensitivity and resolution. High frequency provides better sensitivity to low flow while lower frequency has better penetration and lesser aliasing.

4. Pulse repetition frequency (PRF): called scale: low PRF concerns at low velocities and high PRF reduces aliasing.

5. Area of investigation: larger area reduces frame rate. Thus, reducing the color box of the flow area under examination will usually improve frame rate and may allow a higher color scan line density with improved spatial resolution

6. Focus: should be coincide to the region of interest [2].

2.1.2 Practical guidelines of color Doppler flow imaging

1. Choose the set-up key. This improve Doppler parameters for specific investigations.

2. Apply power within the study area and then adjust color gain. Ensure focus is set at the level of region of investigation. Adjust gain to improve color signal.

3. Position beam steering to get satisfactory beam angle for the selected artery or vein.

4. Adjust PRF to synchronize the flow status. Low PRF are very sensitive to low flows or velocities but may cause aliasing. High PRF decrease aliasing but are less sensitive to low flows/velocities [2].

5. Set the color flow area to suitable size. A small color flow 'box' or region may lead to a better frame rate and better resolution.

2.1.3 Spectral wave Doppler

Pulsed wave Doppler (PWD) ultrasound is used to generate a sonogram of a blood vessel (vein or artery) under study (**Figure 2**). PWD provides a measure of the flow changing velocity throughout the cardiac cycle and display distribution of velocities in the sample volume (gate) as demonstrate in **Figure 3**. Velocities can be measured when an accurate angle correction is made.

2.1.4 Factors affecting the spectral Doppler image

1. Power: set the transmitted power to study area.

2. Gain: influence sensitivity to flow signals.

3. PRF: low PRF is used to detect low velocities while high PRF decrease aliasing.

4. Gate size: beam steering allows improved beam angle for accuracy of calculation of flow velocity.

2.1.5 Guidelines for practical spectral Doppler image

1. Set power to the selected study area.

2. Place the Doppler cursor on the artery/vein to be examined.

3. Gain should be adjusted so that the image is clearly visible and noiseless.

4. Apply the beam steering to get a satisfactory angle. Remember that angles approaching to 90° will give ambiguous image or unclear data. The beam angle must be 60° or less when velocity measurements are to be maintained.

5. Adjust the PRF/scale and baseline to suit flow conditions. The sonogram should be clear and not subjected to aliasing.

6. Adjust the sample volume (SV) to correct and suitable size coincided with area under investigation. Correct the angle to obtain accurate velocities. Use the B-mode and color flow image of the vessel to make the angle correction [2].

2.2 Doppler ultrasound of the kidneys

Doppler ultrasound is essential for evaluation of the kidneys. Doppler is considered more accurate than conventional sonography since it provides functional and

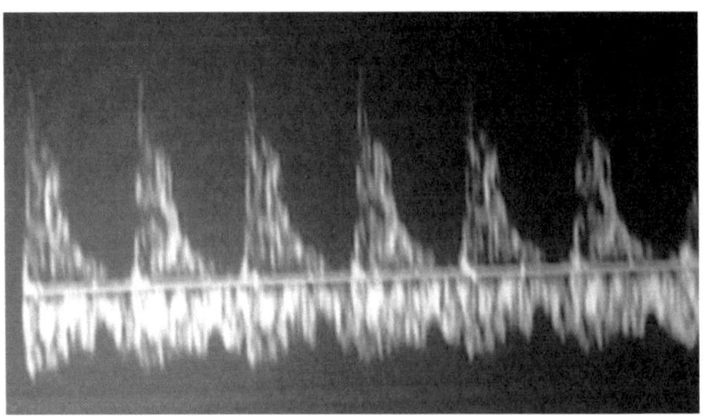

Figure 2.
Spectral wave Doppler. Renal arterial velocity waveform.

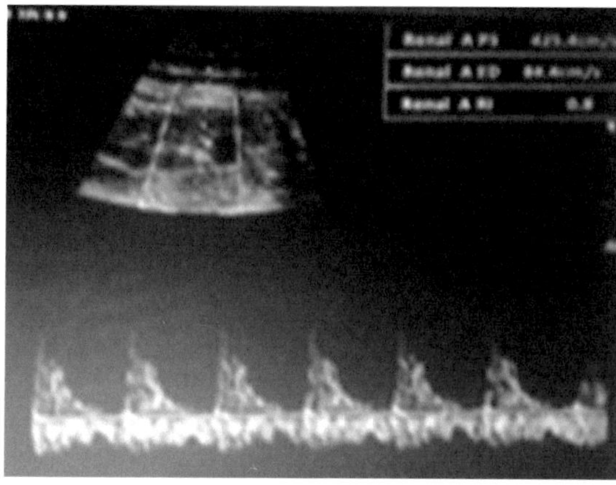

Figure 3.
Renal artery spectral Doppler demonstrates renal artery stenosis; PSV is 452.4 cm/s, RI= 0.80 in a 25-years male with hypertension and abnormal renal function (the sonogram taken by Dr. Moawia Gameraddin).

vascular information which are lacked in grayscale ultrasound. Doppler ultrasound assesses patterns of renal and extrarenal vascularization [3].

Doppler investigations must be performed properly to gain useful data. It allows information about the presence and direction of blood flow in renal vessels. Renal artery stenosis can be assessed by Doppler indices; resistive index (RI), pulsatility index (PI) and systolic to diastolic ratio (S/D). These indices provide hemodynamic and predictive information regarding the renal arteries. Analysis of the RI may provide helpful clinical information in various renal diseases [3].

2.2.1 Doppler procedure of the renal arteries

The investigation starts with the patient in the supine position using a low-frequency probe (2.5–5.0 MHz) to depict the abdominal aorta (AA) and renal arteries (RAs). The two main approaches for imaging the renal arteries are through the anterior abdominal wall. In most situations the anterior approach is used to assess the main RAs [4, 5].

The RAs arise from the lateral borders of the abdominal aorta (AA) at the level of the second lumbar vertebra, almost 1–2 cm inferior to the superior mesenteric artery (SMA) origin. The right RA arises from the anterolateral aspect of the abdominal aorta and it courses under the inferior vena cava (IVC) [8–10]. From this view, RA flow is in a direction that is parallel to the Doppler beam, optimizing signal reception. The patient usually needs to be placed in the opposite lateral decubitus position [4, 6].

A 3.5 MHz curvilinear array transducer with variable focal zone are used. The Doppler examination is usually performed in supine positions as stated by the renal ultrasound protocols. Each Kidney will be examined firstly with B-mode ultrasound in at least two planes to maintain the renal length for each kidney. The Doppler indices (RI and PI) are measured at interlobular or arcuate artery in the upper, middle, and lower portions of the kidney and the mean values were calculated for each kidney.

2.2.2 Normal vascularity of the renal artery

Doppler RI is efficient to detect intrarenal vascular pathological processes. Several studies have demonstrated that a normal mean renal RI is approximately 0.60. It was reported that a mean RI of 0.60 ± 0.01 for individuals without pre-existing renal disease [7]. Other studies also reported normal mean RI values of 0.64 ± 0.05, 0.58 ± 0.05 [8], and 0.62 ± 0.04 [8, 9]. In addition, most sonographers have considered 0.70 to be the upper threshold of the normal RI in adults [10, 11].

2.2.3 The importance of Doppler resistive index

Doppler sonographic analysis of renal artery waveforms was empirically applied to disease characterization (**Figure 4**). Despite RI is a good predictor of several renal abnormalities, there are factors that affect the arterial waveform such as vascular resistance, vascular compliance, and heart rate. In a previous study, it was reported that renal RI was associated with "histological changes and poor renal outcome during chronic kidney disease". It was shown that RI ≥ 0.65 is associated with arteriosclerosis, severe interstitial fibrosis and renal function decline. Therefore, RI is essential Doppler parameter that contribute to diagnose patients at high risk of end-stage renal disease (ESRD) [12].

2.2.4 Application of Doppler in renal diseases

2.2.4.1 The role of Doppler in hypertension

Hypertension involves approximately 25–30% of the adult population and it was reported that the prevalence will increase. It is considered a main risk factor for the development of renal failure and cardiovascular disease. It was reported that 80% of patients with chronic kidney disease (CKD) are hypertensive. The relationship between hypertension and kidney disease is complex and it is attributed to the interrelated pathophysiology. Renal hypertension or renovascular hypertension means hypertension due to renal artery stenosis and kidney disease. Thus, patients who newly diagnosed hypertension must be screened for underlying kidney disease [13].

2.2.4.2 The role of Doppler RI in renal hypertension

The Doppler RI has been utilized for many years in a variety of clinical situations. Doppler ultrasonography detects renal abnormalities at macrovascular and microvascular levels. Assessment of renal RI at different regions of the renal parenchyma may suggest physiological or morphological changes within the kidneys. Therefore, it provides useful information for diagnosis and prognosis of the disease.

Recent studies revealed an increased renal resistive index (RRI) in patients with primary hypertension not only reflects vascular changes in intrarenal supply, but that it is also associated with atherosclerosis and systemic hemodynamics. Therefore, it provides useful prognostic information.

2.2.5 Doppler assessment of non-obstructive diseases

2.2.5.1 Acute and chronic kidney disease

Acute kidney injury: Acute kidney injury (AKI) was reported to associate with a high morbidity, long-term mortality and apparent economic impact [14].

Doppler ultrasound has been widely used in the assessment of renal diseases for diagnosis, prognosis and management. Doppler ultrasound is non-invasive, low cost and safe method for the evaluation of the renal blood flow. Recent studies reported different incidence of AKD among hospitalized patients classified as

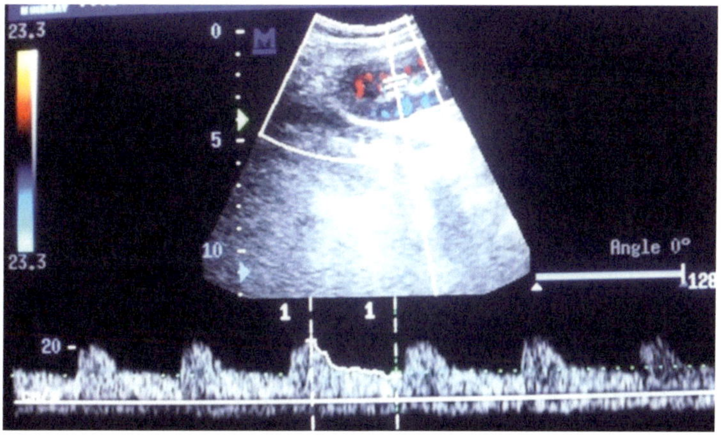

Figure 4.
Duplex Doppler reveals normal waveform of the renal artery (a sonogram taken from Awadia Gareeballah and Moawia Gameraddin researches).

"KDIGO classification (18.3 %), followed by AKIN (16.6 %) and RIFLE (16.1 %) and CK (7.0 %)."

2.2.5.2 Doppler evaluation of acute kidney injury

In gray scale ultrasound, AKD reveals increased renal parenchymal echogenicity which attributed to inflammatory states (acute glomerulonephritis, acute interstitial nephritis, acute tubular necrosis, HIV nephropathy) or infiltrative diseases (lymphoma, monoclonal, myeloma and gammopathies) decreased thickening of kidney cortex and echogenicity are also significant findings of AKI [15]. Color Doppler identifies the renal vessels localization to calculate RRI to monitor renal perfusion. In late stages of AKI, RRI usually exceed 0.7, and a threshold of 0.75 is reported as optimal in recognizing between renal and prerenal disease. However, RRI values lower than 0.7 are related to a good recovery after fluid rehydration, while RRI >0.7 suggest a developing ischemic acute tubular necrosis (ATN) and worse prognosis [16]. In conclusion, RRI play an effective role in different types of AKI.

2.2.6 Doppler assessment of chronic kidney disease

Chronic kidney disease (CKD) is considered as one of the public health problems worldwide [17]. According to the report of Global Burden of Disease in 2010 [2], CKD had been ranked the first cause of death worldwide at 27th to 18th over two decades. It was reported that "the surge of the CKD epidemic over these decades produced an 82% increase in years of life lost related to CKD, a disease toll of the same magnitude of that attributable to diabetes".

Ultrasonography of the kidneys is essential imaging modality among other renal imaging methods since it is available, low cost and safe. US can easily assess a CKD by measuring the length of the kidneys and evaluating the echogenicity of the kidney cortex. The reduction of size and increased echogenicity reflect pathological processes within the kidney.

The normal kidney length is about 11–12 cm (the left kidney is about 3 mm longer than the right kidney) in younger adults and a progressive atrophy with aging. Normal kidney is always as bright as normal liver or spleen tissue [18]. When the kidney cortex became brighter (echogenic) than hepatic tissue or splenic tissue, this reflects inflammatory changes in the kidney tissues. CKD is often associated with increased echogenicity of the renal cortex since fibrous tissue such as glomerulosclerosis interstitial fibrosis, increases echogenicity.

However, those inflammatory conditions such as glomerulonephritis and acute interstitial nephritis (ATN) are associated with hyperechoic aspect of the renal parenchyma. In most cases, small and echogenic kidneys always suggest CKD instead of AKI.

Doppler ultrasound plays effective role in defining CKD and its progression to ESRD. Renal RI is reported to be correlated with arteriolosclerosis, glomerulosclerosis and tubulointerstitial lesions more than others morphologic parameters like kidney length and cortex area [19]. In general, higher values of renal RI (>0.7) ordinary reflects more severe arteriolosclerosis than normal values (<0.65) or high normal RRI ($0.65 \leq RI < 0.7$) [20]. However, patients with high-normal renal RI revealed good response to steroid therapy compared to a RRI > 0.7 [19]. Additionally, patients with advanced CKD stage showed significant higher RI than patients with earlier CKD stage.

2.2.7 Renal masses

Ultrasound plays a key role in screening renal cancer in asymptomatic patients. Most renal tumors remain are not accurately diagnosed on US and require CT for further characterization. However, US help to characterize cystic RCC that remain unclear on computerize tomography (CT). Recent technology in gray-scale imaging have improved the accuracy of US in the diagnosis and staging of kidney cancer. In addition, solid renal masses can grossly be categorized as completely solid, multifocal, or partially cystic tumors. The cystic appearance is mainly due to necrosis.

2.2.7.1 Ultrasound evaluation kidney cancer

Computed tomography (CT) is the gold standard for imaging the kidneys. It is accurate for detecting and characterizing renal neoplasms and staging renal cell carcinoma (RCC). On the other hand, ultrasound (US) has a less sensitivity in detecting small renal lesions, but it plays a key role in the early diagnosis of kidney cancer since it is routinely used in the evaluation of the abdomen. Renal masses were identified on US as a distortion of the normal tissue echotexture. Previous studies reported that RCC is detected incidentally in asymptomatic patients. Only 10% of patients with RCC present with the classic triad of hematuria, pain and a flank mass. Most of these patients often have advanced disease. More than 40% of the present with none of these three symptoms [21]. The RCC might be detected incidentally during abdominal sonography. The majority of RCC measure less than 3 cm or less on US. Early detection of RCC improves prognosis and survival rate.

The sonographic appearance of renal tumors vary between isoechoic-, hypoechoic, and hyperechoic compared with the normal renal parenchyma [22]. Doppler US assesses the blood flow patterns of vascularity in renal tumor tissue. It reveals vessels with high velocities. In RCC, the hypervascularity is attributed to neovascularization. The Doppler RI on spectral Doppler US was reported to be useful in detecting RCC in patients with ESRD [23].

2.2.8 The Doppler assessment of transplanted kidney

US is the most imaging modality for assessment of the transplanted kidneys (TK) (**Figure 5**). The TR is located in the right or left iliac fossa. The superficial location of the graft make the US examination accurate and ideal. The renal graft

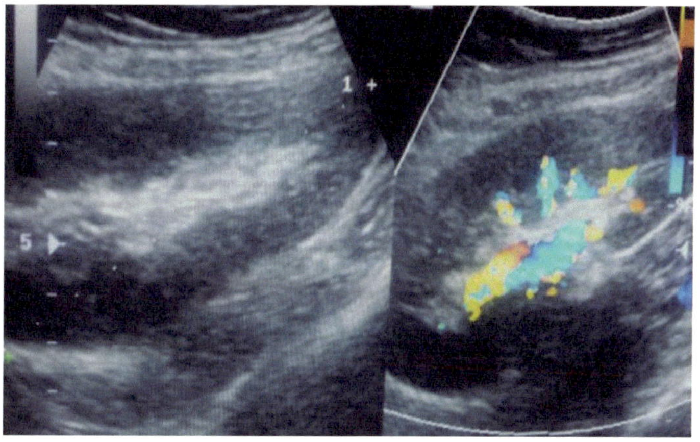

Figure 5.
A sonogram of a transplanted kidney shows normal size and normal color flow.

is vulnerable to several pathologic changes which might occur immediately or later. The sonographic appearance for evaluation of immediate post-plant pathologies may not be specific such as acute tubular necrosis (ATN), acute rejection, and toxicity associated with immunosuppressive calcineurin inhibitors [24].

The Doppler renal RI has a significant correlation with renal allograft size. It was reported that RI of 0.8 or higher was considered a strong predictor of graft failure and morphological changes [25]. The increase of RI was reported to correlate with presence of acute rejection and ATN [26]. On the other hand, elevated serum creatinine levels in renal transplant patient reveals high RI values. Therefore, the renal RI was a good predictor of graft function.

3. Renal elastography

Ultrasound elastography (USE) was first described in the 1990s. It is an imaging technology which is sensitive to tissue stiffness. In recent years, elastography has been further developed to enable quantitative assessments of tissue stiffness. Elastography is capable to assess changed elasticity of soft tissues resulting from specific pathological or physiological processes [27]. For example, tissue of solid tumors tends to differ mechanically from surrounding healthy tissues. Furthermore, fibrosis makes diseased tissue to be stiffer than normal ones. The role of elastography is to differentiate diseased tissue from normal one for diagnostic applications.

Ultrasound elastography (USE) of the kidneys is a potential application is an advanced imaging tool that may become a clinical biomarker for disease. However, elastography of renal transplant cortex and the corticomedullary strain ratio have been studied and they were found to correlate with renal cortical fibrosis [28, 29]. Shear-wave elastography (SWE) of the kidney utilizing acoustic radiation force impulse (ARFI) is a potential clinical application which was reported to demonstrate successful clinical applications in human organs [29]. In the kidney, SWE has shown promise in the evaluation of CKD, renal transplant function, and renal vein thrombosis (RVT).

3.1 Renal fibrosis

USE is clinically useful to detect and assess fibrosis in CKD and transplanted kidneys. USE with both strain imaging and SWI methods are noninvasively to

Criteria	Doppler ultrasound	Elastography
Main principle	Evaluates vascularity	Assesses elasticity
Renal transplantation	Renal blood resistivity index (renal RI) above 0.8 indicates renal graft dysfunction.	Assesses cortical fibrosis in early stage. Additionally, elastography assesses the grades of fibrosis; distinguish mild from moderate fibrosis.
Obstructive and non-obstructive hydronephrosis	Doppler US distinguishes between obstructive and non-obstructive hydronephrosis. Obstructive hydronephrosis reveals higher RI values than non-obstructive hydronephrosis.	Measurements did not enable distinguishing of obstructive hydronephrosis from non-obstructive hydronephrosis in children
Differentiation between malignant and benign tumors	Doppler US is useful in characterization of renal pseudotumors. Doppler allows differentiation of normal vascularity from tumor neovascularity. On the other hand, benign renal masses characterized by less or peripheral vascularity, homogeneous echotextures and well-defined margins.	Malignant tumors are stiffer than benign masses.

Table 1.
Comparison between Doppler ultrasound and elastography in evaluation of abnormalities of the kidney.

detect, stage and monitor kidney fibrosis, thus, reducing the need for renal biopsy [30]. SWI is preferable to strain imaging in evaluating kidney fibrosis in both renal graft and native kidneys since it is independent of external compression [30]. A previous study reported that SWE renal stiffness was higher in patients affected with CKD than in healthy controls [31]. Therefore, tissue stiffness measured by USE was significantly correlated with histopathologic renal fibrosis. This finding concluded that, USE is a non-invasive tool for predicting kidney fibrosis.

3.2 Characterization of focal renal lesions using elastography

USE is useful for characterizing focal renal masses since US features are not specific for malignancy. Assessment of renal masses with USE have shown controversial results. Some results found SW velocity values could differentiate between benign and malignant masses. Another study compared between malignant and benign renal masses concluded that malignant tumors are 2.8 times stiffer than benign masses [32]. A previous study reported that USE can differentiate between renal cell carcinoma (RCC) and transitional cell carcinoma (TCC) [33]. In general, quantification of kidney tissue using USE is more complex than other organs since the high heterogeneity of the renal tissue. However, the combination of doppler ultrasound and elastography will provide better assessment of kidney abnormalities as compared in **Table 1**.

4. Conclusion

In summary, Doppler ultrasound and USE are very effective imaging method to the kidneys. Doppler assesses vascularity of the kidneys while elastography evaluates tissue elasticity. USE is a new developing method and various studies have been made using elastography in kidneys. It is very effective on the transplanted and CKD kidneys to evaluate the corticomedullary fibrosis to prevent invasive biopsy.

Conflict of interest

The author declares there was no conflict of interest regarding this chapter.

Author details

Moawia Gameraddin
Department of Diagnostic Radiologic Technology, Faculty of Applied Medical Sciences, Taibah University, Almadinah, Kingdom of Saudi Arabia

*Address all correspondence to: gameraldinm@gmail.com

References

[1] Hansen KL, Nielsen MB, Ewertsen C. Ultrasonography of the kidney: A pictorial review. Diagnostics (Basel). 2015;**6**(1):2. DOI: 10.3390/diagnostics6010002

[2] Available from: https://sonoworld.com/client/fetus/html/doppler/capitulos-html/chapter_01.htm [Accessed: 27 Jan. 2019]

[3] Granata A, Fiorini F, Andrulli S, et al. Doppler ultrasound and renal artery stenosis: An overview. Journal of Ultrasound. 2009;**12**(4):133-143

[4] Zubarev AV. Ultrasound of renal vessels. European Radiology. 2001;**11**:1902-1915

[5] Meola M, Petrucci I. Color Doppler sonography in the study of chronic ischemic nephropathy. Journal of Ultrasound. 2008;**11**(2):55-73

[6] Korst MB, Joosten FB, Postma CT, Jager GJ, Krabbe JK, Barentsz JO. Accuracy of normal-dose contrast-enhanced MR angiography in assessing renal artery stenosis and accessory renal artery stenosis and accessory renal arteries. American Journal of Roentgenology. 2000;**174**:629-634. [PubMed]

[7] Keogan M, Kliewer M, Hertzberg B, DeLong DM, Tupler RH, Carroll BA. Renal resistive indexes: Variability in Doppler US measurement in a healthy population. Radiology. 1996;**199**:165-169

[8] Norris C, Pfeiffer J, Rittgers S, Barnes RW. Noninvasive evaluation of renal artery stenosis and renovascular resistance: Experimental and clinical studies. J Vasc Surg. 1984;**1**:192-201

[9] Kim S, Kim W, Choi B, Kim CW. Duplex sonography of the native kidney: Resistive index vs serum creatinine. (abstract). Journal of Ultrasound in Medicine. 1990;**9**:S25

[10] Platt J, Ellis J, Rubin J. Examination of native kidneys with duplex Doppler ultrasound. Seminars in Ultrasound, CT, and MR. 1991;**12**:308-318

[11] Platt J. Doppler evaluation of native kidney dysfunction: Obstructive and nonobstructive disease. AJR. 1992;**158**:1035-1042

[12] Bigé N, Lévy PP, Callard P, et al. Renal arterial resistive index is associated with severe histological changes and poor renal outcome during chronic kidney disease. BMC Nephrology. 2012;**13**:139. DOI: 10.1186/1471-2369-13-139

[13] Grendelmeier I. Renal hypertension—The role of the kidneys in blood pressure regulation and the kidneys as end-organ. Therapeutische Umschau. 2015;**72**(6):369-374. DOI: 10.1024/0040-5930/a000688

[14] Nisula S, Kaukonen KM, Vaara ST, Korhonen AM, Poukkanen M, Karlsson S, et al. Intensive Care Medicine. 2013;**39**:420-428. DOI: 10.1007/s00134-012-2796-5

[15] Legrand MM, Darmon M. Renal imaging in acute kidney injury. In: Acute Nephrology for the Critical Care Physician. 2015

[16] Pozzi Mucelli R, Bertolotto M, Quaia E. Imaging techniques in acute renal failure. Contributions to Nephrology. 2001;**132**:76-91. DOI: 10.1159/000060076

[17] Neuen BL, Chadban SJ, Demaio AR, Johnson DW, Perkovic V. Chronic kidney disease and the global NCDs agenda. BMJ Global Health.

2017;**2**(2):e000380. DOI: 10.1136/bmjgh-2017-000380

[18] Spatola L, Andrulli S. Doppler ultrasound in kidney diseases: A key parameter in clinical long-term follow-up. Journal of Ultrasound. 2016;**19**:243-250

[19] Hanamura K, Tojo A, Knugasa S, Asaba K, Fujita TT. The resistive index is a marker of renal function, pathology, prognosis, and responsiveness to steroid therapy in chronic kidney disease patients. International Journal of Nephrology. 2012;**2012**:139565

[20] Gibbons RP, Monte JE, Correa RJ Jr, Mason JT. Manifestations of renal cell carcinoma. Urology. 1976;**8**:201-206

[21] Ikee R, Kobayashi S, Hemmi N, et al. Correlation between the resistive index by Doppler ultrasound and kidney function and histology. American Journal of Kidney Diseases. 2005;**46**(4):603-609

[22] Rumack CM, Wilson SR, Charboneau JW, Levine D. Diagnostic Ultrasound. St Louis, MO, USA: Elsevier Health Sciences; 2005

[23] Kim SY, Woo S, Hwang SI, et al. Usefulness of resistive index on spectral Doppler ultrasonography in the detection of renal cell carcinoma in patients with end-stage renal disease. Ultrasonography. 2014;**33**(2):136-142

[24] Piyasena RV, Hamper UM. Doppler evaluation of renal transplants. Applied Radiology. Available from: https://www.appliedradiology.com/articles/doppler-ultrasound-evaluation-of-renal-transplants [Accessed: 20 Jan. 2019]

[25] Gameradin M, Malik BA, Yousef M, Gareeballah A, Siddig S, Burai M, et al. Renal transplantation: Sonography and Doppler assessment of transplanted kidneys in adult Sudanese patients. Australasian Medical Journal. 2017;**10**(6):489-496. DOI: 10.21767/AMJ.2017.2994

[26] Radermacher J, Mengel M, Ellis S. The renal arterial resistance index and renal allograft survival. The New England Journal of Medicine. 2003;**349**:115-124

[27] Shiina T, Nightingale KR, Palmeri ML, Hall TJ, Bamber JC, Barr RG, et al. WFUMB guidelines and recommendations for clinical use of ultrasound elastography: Part 1: Basic principles and terminology. Ultrasound in Medicine & Biology. 2015;**41**:1126-1147

[28] Gao J, Weitzel W, Rubin JM, Hamilton J, Lee J, Dadhania D, et al. Renal transplant elasticity ultrasound imaging: Correlation between normalized strain and renal cortical fibrosis. Ultrasound in Medicine & Biology. 2013;**39**:1536-1542

[29] Gao J, Min R, Hamilton J, Weitzel W, Chen J, Juluru K, et al. Corticomedullary strain ratio: A quantitative marker for assessment of renal allograft cortical fibrosis. Journal of Ultrasound in Medicine. 2013;**32**:1769-1775

[30] Anvari A, Barr RG, Dhyani M, Samir AE. Clinical application of sonoelastography in thyroid, prostate, kidney, pancreas, and deep venous thrombosis. Abdominal Imaging. 2015;**40**:709-722

[31] Samir AE, Allegretti AS, Zhu Q, et al. Shear wave elastography in chronic kidney disease: A pilot experience in native kidneys. BMC Nephrology. 2015;**16**:119. DOI: 10.1186/s12882-015-0120-7

[32] Onur MR, Poyraz AK, Bozgeyik Z, Onur AR, Orhan I. Utility of

semiquantitative strain elastography for differentiation between benign and malignant solid renal masses. Journal of Ultrasound in Medicine. 2015;**34**:639-647

[33] Inci MF, Kalayci TO, Tan S, Karasu S, Albayrak E, Cakir V, et al. Diagnostic value of strain elastography for differentiation between renal cell carcinoma and transitional cell carcinoma of kidney. Abdominal Radiology (NY). 2016;**41**(6):1152-1159. DOI: 10.1007/s00261-016-0658-2

Section 6

Intestinal Ultrasound

Chapter 6

High-Frequency Ultrasound Imaging of the Intestine in Normal Subjects and Patients with Intestinal Parasites

Philip C. Njemanze, Josephine T. Njemanze, Clara C. Ofoegbu, Chinwendu C. Darlington, Esther Nneke, Ijeoma A. Onweni, Uchechi V. Ejiogu, Chinenye U. Mgbenu, Nneoma E. Ukeje, Anthonia C. Amadi and Doris C. Amaefule

Abstract

High-frequency ultrasound imaging was used to evaluate the intestinal walls of the duodenum and colon in patients with intestinal parasitic infections. Ultrasound images were obtained from 100 consecutive patients with symptomatic intestinal parasitic diseases and 40 healthy controls. High-frequency annular array transducer of 7.5 MHz was used to obtain B-mode ultrasound gray-scale and color images of the duodenum and colon with and without water contrast. The diagnosis of parasitic infections was based on clinical presentation, serial stool microscopy, and finding of parasites in duodenal aspirates. We demonstrated normal duodenum and colon echoanatomy in control subjects. In patients with giardiasis, the lesions of the duodenum and colon were associated with increased dimensions and wall thickness compared to healthy controls ($p < 0.05$). The ultrasound features of giardial lesions were characterized by increased wall echogenicity, flattening or loss of duodenal folds, and/or colonic haustration, hyperechoic floating foci demonstrating chaotic motility, increased perilesional tissue echogenicity, and altered colonic peristalsis. In amebic lesions there were hyperechoic floating foci with bulk motility. There is loss of wall thickness at amebic ulcer sites or wall thickening at amebic granuloma. Helminths were visualized as large hyperechoic linear or curvilinear foci with serpentine or jolting motility. In conclusion, high-frequency B-mode ultrasound imaging with water contrast demonstrated details of duodenal and colonic echoanatomy in normal subjects and patients with giardiasis.

Keywords: parasites, diarrhea, tropical diseases, water-borne diseases, gastrointestinal tract

1. Introduction: clinical problem

Intestinal parasites infect over three billion people [1]. An intestinal parasite is an organism that lives in the intestine of the host and gets its food from its host.

There are two main classes of parasites that infect the human intestine: protozoa and helminthes [2].

1.1 Intestinal protozoa

Intestinal protozoa are microscopic unicellular organisms that could be free-living or parasitic within the intestine. It could be transmitted from human-to-human through fecal-oral route usually through contaminated food or water, or person-to-person contact [2].

The intestinal protozoa are classified according to motility as:

a. Sarcodina—*Amoeba* (e.g., Entamoeba)

b. Mastigophora—flagellates (e.g., *Giardia*)

c. Ciliophora—ciliates (e.g., *Balantidium*)

1.2 Intestinal helminthes

Intestinal helminthes are macroscopic large, multi-cellular organisms that are visible to the naked eye in adult stage in free-living or parasitic condition in the intestine [2].

There are three main groups of human intestinal helminthes:

1. Platyhelminths or flatworms include trematodes (flukes) and cestodes (tapeworms, e.g., *Taenia saginata*).

2. Thorny-headed worms (acanthocephalins) that infect the intestine in humans.

3. Roundworms include nematodes (e.g., *Ancylostoma duodenale* and *Ascaris lumbricoides*) in which adult forms infect the intestine.

2. Ultrasound classification of features of intestinal parasites

The use of ultrasound to study the features of intestinal parasites has been referred to as high-frequency ultrasound duodenography and colonography with and without water contrast [3, 4]. The ultrasound classification of the features of intestinal parasites is based on:

1. Ultrasonic reflector

2. Hyperechoicity

3. Motility

4. Changes in intestinal wall thickness.

2.1 Ultrasonic reflector

1. Directly visible parasites—e.g., Helminths

2. Indirectly visible parasites on "floaters" (formed by intestinal inclusions)—e.g., *Amoeba* and *Giardia*.

2.2 Hyperechoicity

1. Hyperechoic floating foci (HFF) showing small echogenic particles in floatation, e.g., *Giardia*.

2. Hyperechoic curvilinear foci show a large echogenic curved and/or linear independent objects, e.g., *Ascaris*.

2.3 Motility

1. Bulk motility by slow active movement of the large mass of the lesion at the same time in the same direction independent of gastrointestinal motility—e.g., *Amoeba*.

2. Chaotic motility by fast active movement of singular or small groups of the lesion in different directions independent of gastrointestinal motility, e.g., *Giardia* and *Balantinum*.

3. Jolting motility by fast jerks, e.g. *Ancylostoma*.

4. Serpentine motility by serpentine-like movement, e.g. *Ascariasis*.

2.4 Changes in intestinal wall thickness

1. Increased wall thickening of all layers by cystoskeletal dysfunction, e.g., *Giardia*.

2. Increased wall thickening by abscess formation, e.g., *Amoeba*.

3. No change in wall thickness, e.g., helminths.

4. Loss of tri-layer wall replaced by single layer due to cytoskeletal rearrangement caused by multiple parasitic lesions in immune-compromised patients (e.g., giardiasis in patients with HIV/AIDS).

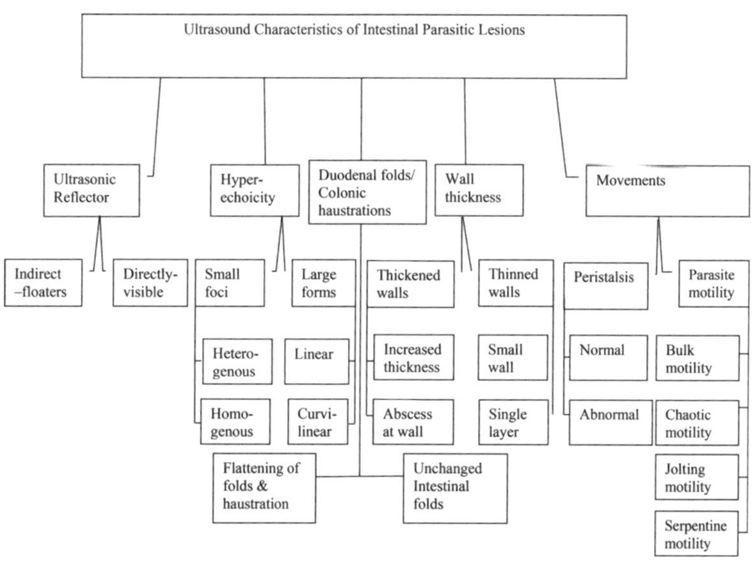

Figure 1.
Schematic diagram of the classification based on ultrasound imaging features of intestinal parasites.

2.5 Changes in duodenal folds and colonic haustrations

1. Flattening of duodenal folds and colonic haustrations, e.g., *Giardia*.

2. Thinning of duodenal folds and colonic haustrations, e.g., *Giardia* in immune compromised patients.

3. Thickening of duodenal folds and colonic haustrations, e.g., advanced disease in giardiasis and amebiasis.

Figure 1 shows the schematic diagram for ultrasonic characterization of the lesions caused by the different types of common intestinal parasites (protozoan and helminthes).

3. Technique of high-frequency ultrasound duodenography and colonography

3.1 Patient examination

To evaluate the intestine, patient preparation is needed. All ultrasound examinations are performed with and without water contrast after overnight fasting (for at least 16 h) using standard scanning procedure [4]. Water contrast imaging is performed by having adult subjects take at least 1 L of water prior to examination. Subject examination is performed in the supine horizontal, left-posterior oblique, and left-lateral decubitus positions using the intercostal and subcostal approaches. The internal organs, including liver, gall bladder, spleen, pancreas, duodenum, colon, and kidneys, are routinely evaluated in all subjects. The abdominal ultrasound examination are performed using B-mode and color flow Doppler ultrasonography with 2.5 and 7.5 MHz annular array transducers of a duplex color flow Doppler ultrasound system (Agilent HP/Philips SONOS 5500, Philips Medical Systems, Cambridge, MA, USA). The examination begins with deeply located abdominal structures using 2.5 MHz probe. The detailed examination of duodenal walls and folds is performed using 7.5 MHz probe beginning in the right hypochondriac (1) and epigastric (2) regions (see **Figure 2**). This is followed by the examination of the colonic walls and haustra [3, 4] of the ascending colon starting from the McBurney's point that lies one-third of the distance laterally on a line drawn from the umbilicus to the right anterior superior iliac spine. The examination proceeds upward to the right lumbar (4), right hypochondriac (1), and turning clockwise to the epigastric (2), left-hypochondriac (3), left-lumbar (6), and left-iliac (9) regions (see **Figure 2**).

Color flow Doppler sonography is performed to examine the localization of lesions in relation to vessels and body abdominal cavities. All ultrasound studies including measurements and grading of echogenicity are performed by a trained sonographer using built-in software [4]. Measurements are taken between peristaltic waves on a water contrast image.

3.2 Sonographic findings in normal duodenum

The duodenal wall is visualized as alternate bands of moderately echogenic mucosa with hyperechoic core submucosa which are thrown into folds of Kerckring, arranged circularly, a middle hypoechoic muscularis layer and an outer hyperechoic serosa layer [3, 4]. **Figure 3** shows the measurement end-points including wall thickness in the duodenum (with water contrast) (**Figure 3**; within double blue arrow ends), measured between two mucosal folds of Kerckring [4] (**Figure 3**; white arrow heads), from the surface of the moderately echogenic mucosa, through the hyperechoic submucosa (**Figure 3**; red arrow) and hypoechoic muscularis (**Figure 3**; within double brown arrow ends) to the hyperechoic serosa layer (**Figure 2**; bottom red arrow head). The wall thickness of the duodenum is 3.5 ± 2.2 mm [4].

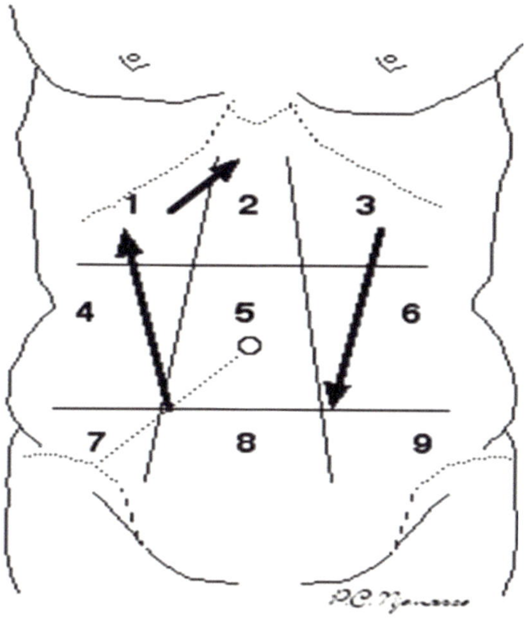

Figure 2.
Locations for placement of transducer for examination of the intestine.

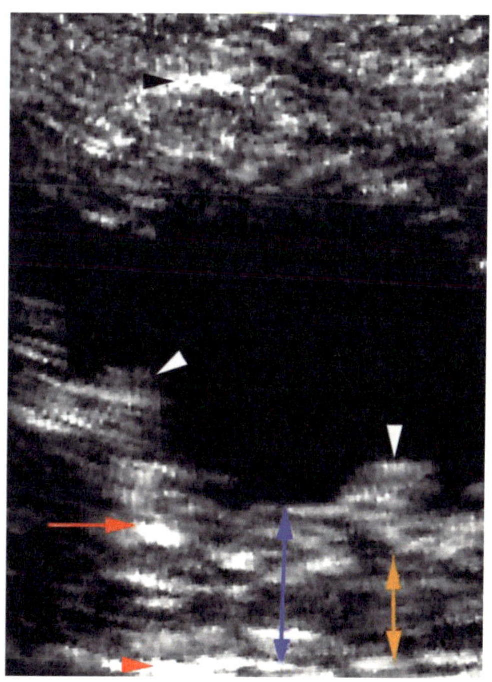

Figure 3.
Measurement end-points of the duodenum with water contrast.

3.3 Sonographic findings in normal colon

Figure 4A shows the colonic wall comprising alternate hypoechoic and hyperechoic bands corresponding to the histological layers. The latter comprises a moderately echogenic mucosa, a hyperechoic core submucosa, a hypoechoic muscularis layer, and an outer hyperechoic serosa [3, 4]. The outer layer of the longitudinal muscle in the colon demonstrated a relatively hyperechoic *tenia coli librae*. The haustra are isoechoic with the mucosa. The wall thickness of the colon (**Figure 4A**; with water contrast), (**Figure 4A**; within double blue arrow ends) is measured between two haustra (**Figure 4A**; white arrow heads), from the surface of the moderately echogenic mucosa (**Figure 4A**; top arrow of the double blue arrows), through the hyperechoic submucosa (**Figure 4A**; brown arrow), and hypoechoic muscularis (**Figure 4A**, within double brown arrow ends) layers, to the hyperechoic serosa layer (**Figure 4A**; bottom brown arrow head); and diameter measurement is taken from near wall serosa (**Figure 4A**; top brown arrow head) to far wall serosa (**Figure 4A**; bottom brown arrow head). The measurement cursor line is aligned perpendicular to the echogenic *tenia coli librae* (**Figure 4A**; cursor line between brown arrow heads) which runs midway between the near and far wall serosa in long axis view of the ascending and descending colon. The ascending colon diameter is 32.0 ± 13.3 mm and wall thickness is 3.9 ± 1.4 mm [4]. The descending colon diameter is 30.7 ± 8.5 mm and wall thickness is 3.8 ± 0.8 mm [4]. **Figure 4B** (white arrows) shows the haustra with pyramidal shape, regular contour, homogenous and spaced at regular intervals [3, 4].

3.4 Normal colonic peristalsis

Colonic peristalsis was observed sonographically in control subjects using real-time images taken with water contrast. Local movements of the colon aid the absorption of water and help to form feces by providing a kneading action. The peristaltic movements are brought about by contractions of segments of circular muscles and

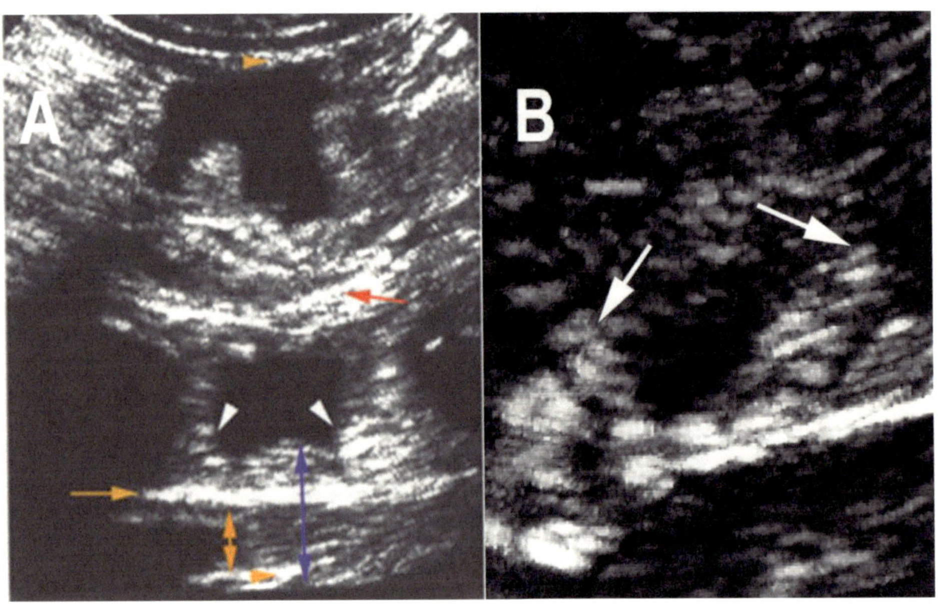

Figure 4.
Measurement end-points in the ascending and descending colon with water contrast (A), and pyramidal shaped haustra in the ascending colon (B, white arrows).

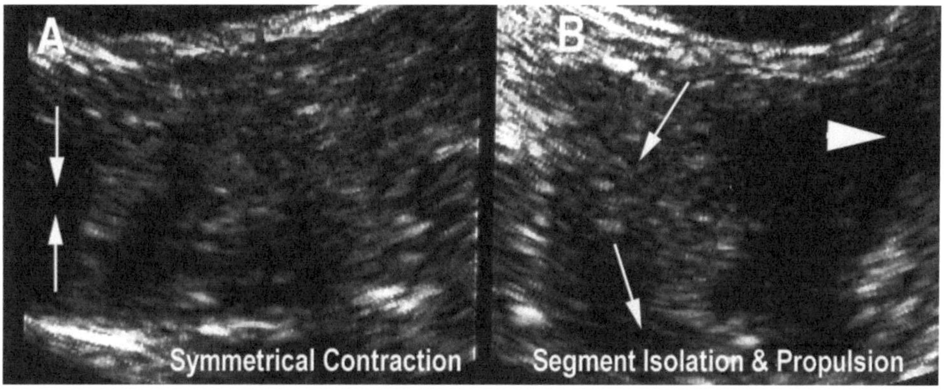

Figure 5.
Normal colonic peristalsis showing symmetrical contraction rings (A, white arrows) that isolate the segments followed by antegrade propulsion of colonic inclusions (B, white arrow head).

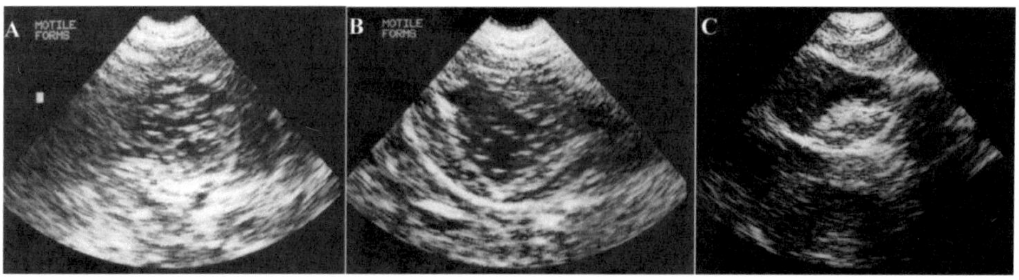

Figure 6.
Shows hyperechoic floating foci within the duodenum without water contrast (A), and with water contrast (B); while there is a condensed hyperechoic foci with bulk motility of Amoeba with water contrast (C).

the adjacent portions of the *tenia coli* [4]. The latter movements are termed segmentations; they produce folds of the wall known as haustra (**Figure 5A**; white arrow heads). During peristalsis, there are circumferential symmetrical contraction rings (**Figure 5A**; white arrows) formed between adjacent haustra, and sequential segment isolation from the rest of the gastrointestinal tract (GIT) followed by antegrade propulsion of content (**Figure 6B**; white arrows) [4]. Contractions of the smooth muscle in the colonic walls produced a rise in intraluminal pressure within the isolated chamber [5, 6]. This is followed by relaxation of one of the two rings enclosing a segment, and results in peristaltic propulsion of the colonic inclusions (**Figure 5B**; white big arrow head). The walls maintain symmetric contours during contraction (**Figure 5A**; white arrows) and relaxation (**Figure 5B**; white arrows) [4].

3.5 Hyperechoic floating foci with chaotic and bulk motility

The parasitic lesions are located in the duodenum and colon and verified by morphology in stool analysis [6–9]. The microscopic protozoan parasites could not be imaged directly with ultrasound, but could be seen indirectly as they float on intestinal inclusions called floaters which reflect the ultrasound waves [10]. The flagellated protozoan *Giardia* appear as hyperechoic small foci on floaters which are either heterogeneous or homogeneous depending on the floater substance without water contrast (**Figure 6A**), and with water contrast (**Figure 6B**) in the duodenum. Giardial lesion imaged with water contrast present as lesser echogenic HFF with chaotic motility, defined as sonographically observed rapid floatation movements in all directions by hyperechoic floating foci, between peristaltic waves (**Figure 6A, B**) [4].

The *Amoeba* with pseudopods on fatty dense floaters are echogenic and move by slow bulk motion en-mass in a given direction in helical fashion (**Figure 6C**) [4, 8]. The fatty substances as floaters are more echogenic without water contrast (**Figure 7A**) than non-fatty substances or after water contrast (**Figure 7B**).

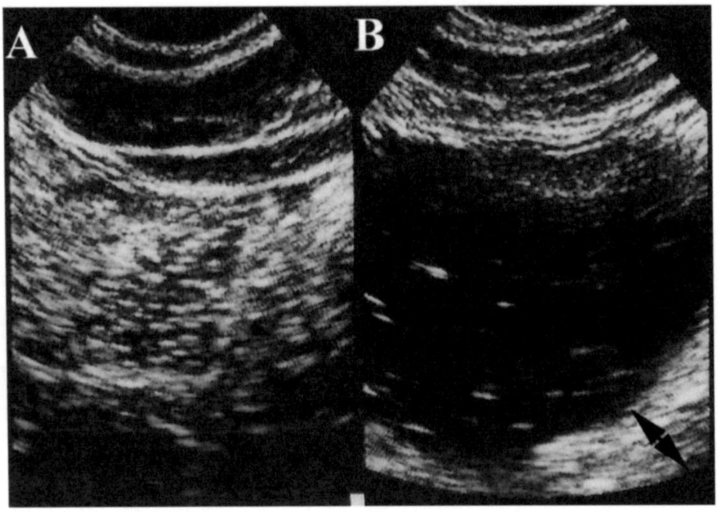

Figure 7.
The ascending colon with hyperechoic floating foci (HFF) without water contrast (A) and with water contrast the image appears hypoechoic (B). The HFF display fast chaotic motility by the flagellated Giardia on floaters.

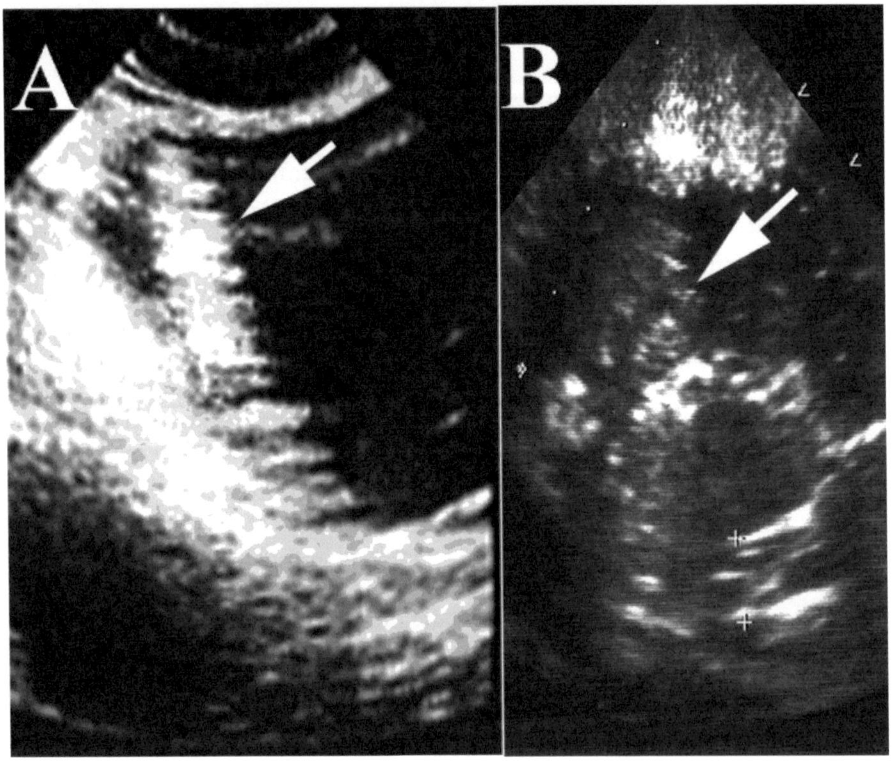

Figure 8.
Helminths parasites as large hyperechoic linear form as seen with Ascaris (A, white arrow) compared to hypercurvilinear form as seen with Taenia (B, white arrow).

3.6 Hyperechoic linear and curvilinear forms with serpentine and jolting motility

The macroscopic helminthic parasites could be visualized directly, and the body parts seen in the reflected ultrasound waves, sometimes with internal details of the gut of the worm. Some parasites may appear as large hyperechoic linear forms (HLF) with rapid spasmodic movement in what could be described as voluntary jolting motility (**Figure 8A**), seen in ascariasis [11, 12]. Other forms of helminthes are hyperechoic curvilinear forms (HCF), which display slow "serpentine" motility (**Figure 8B**), seen in teniasis [13]. The parasites were all identified by morphology in stool analysis.

4. Differential diagnosis

Table 1 shows the differential characteristics of protozoan and helminthic lesions. The protozoan parasites increase wall thickness of the layers and cross-sectional diameter of the duodenum, which occasionally caused flattening of duodenal folds of Kerckring. There is increased wall thickness of the ascending and descending colon of all three layers or at some specific sites due to the presence of amebic abscess [4]. The colonic haustrations are normal in simple infections, but could be flattened in advanced disease. The protozoan HFF could be differentiated by parasite motility. The major differential diagnosis for giardiasis is the ciliated protozoal infection—balantidiasis, that could potentially give rise to HFF. Balantidiasis [14] is caused by a ciliated protozoa—*Balantidium coli*; and is excluded based on clinical, epidemiologic, and laboratory findings. In patients with giardiasis there is absence of history of balantidial dysentery. Amebic lesion demonstrates bulk slow motility as a large mass of the lesion actively moves in one direction at a time. In contrast, giardial lesion demonstrates chaotic motility observed as rapid floatation movements in all directions between peristaltic waves. The helminthic lesion could be differentiated based on size/form and motility. *Ascaris lumbricoides* shows a large hyperechoic linear form (HLF) with jolting motility, different from *Ancylostoma duodenale* which is a relatively small HLF with jolting motility. *Taenia saginata* presents as large hyperechoic curvilinear form with serpentine motility.

4.1 Peculiarities of giardial lesions in the duodenum and colon

Giardial lesions could be distinguished by location, and changes in wall thickness, increased echogenicity of wall tissue, increased cross-sectional diameter, flattening or loss of duodenal folds and/or colonic haustration, presence of HFF with chaotic motility, presence of perilesional tissue echogenicity, and abnormal colonic peristalsis [4]. In patients with giardiasis, the duodenal wall thickness (6.3 ± 1.3 mm) is greater than that in healthy controls (**Figure 9A**, white arrow head), with loss of folds of Kerckring (**Figure 9A**, two white big arrows) and HFF (**Figure 9A**, small white arrow) [4]. In severe disease, the thickness of the duodenal wall could be several times of that seen in normal controls (**Figure 9B**, two white arrow heads), causing compression of adjacent tissues with a thin area of perilesional edema (**Figure 9B**, white arrow) [4].

In symptomatic giardiasis, the wall thickness (8.8 ± 1.4 mm) of the ascending colon is greater than that in healthy controls [3, 4]. Similarly, the wall thickness (9.2 ± 1.2 mm) of the descending colon is greater than that in healthy controls [4]. The increased wall thickness of the ascending colon is best seen with water contrast imaging (**Figure 7A, B**). In immune-compromised patients, giardial lesions could cause thinning of intestinal walls to only a single layer wall (**Figure 9C**) with loss of intestinal haustrations and folds (**Figure 9D**) [4].

Differential diagnosis based on ultrasound characteristics of intestinal parasites

Group of parasite	Genus	Locomotion	Ultrasonic reflector	Duodenal folds/ haustrations	Wall thickness	Hyperechoicity	Lesion motility	Intestinal peristalsis
Protozoan	*Giardia*	Flagellates	Floaters	Flattening in advanced diseases	Thickened walls	Small foci	Chaotic motility	Abnormal retropulsion
	Amoebida	Pseudopods	Floaters	Loss at amebic ulcer sites	Amebic granuloma	Small foci	Bulk motility	Abnormal
Helminths	*Ascaris*	Serpentine	Parasite body part large	Normal	Normal	Large linear form	Jolting motility	Normal
	Taenia	Serpentine	Parasite body part is large	Normal	Normal	Large curvilinear form	Serpentine motility	Normal
	Ancylostoma	Serpentine	Parasite body part is small	Normal	Normal	Small linear form	Jolting motility	Normal

Table 1.
Differential diagnosis of protozoa and helminthes intestinal parasites.

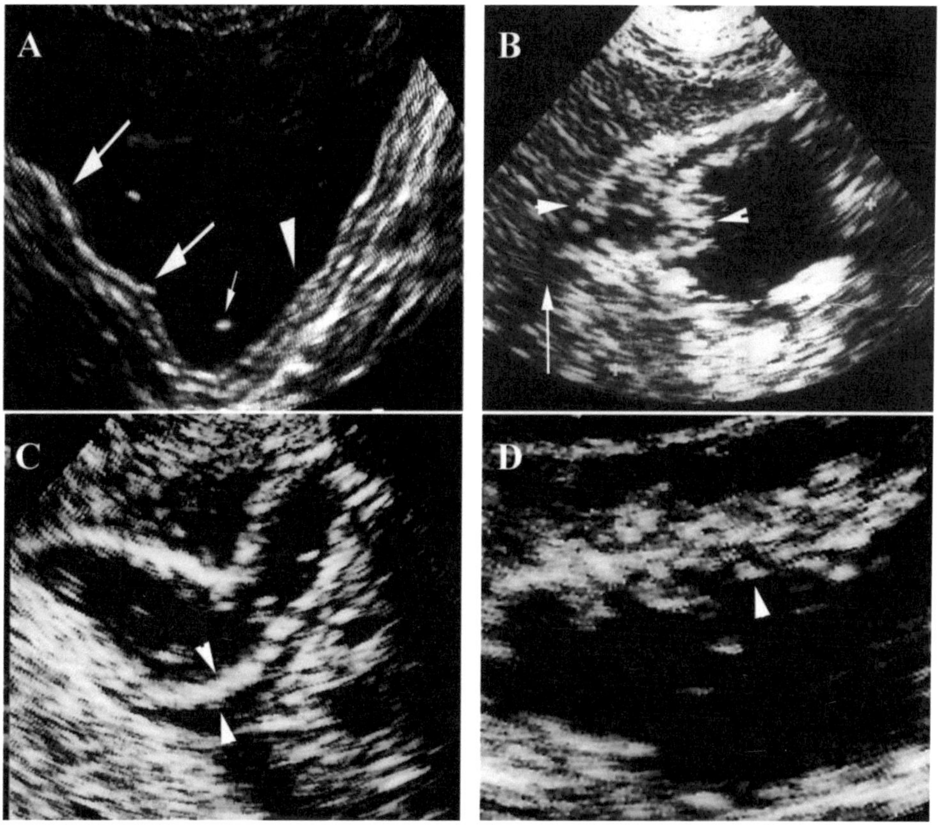

Figure 9.
Severe giardial lesions may cause duodenal wall thickening (A) with loss of folds, and in some cases there may be increased wall thickness (B). In immune-compromised patients there could be thinning of the intestinal wall to a single layer (C), and loss of colonic haustrations (D).

4.2 Abnormal colonic peristalsis in giardiasis

Colonic peristalsis could be observed sonographically with water contrast. The colon demonstrates circumferential asymmetric contraction rings that stretch the wall more on one end than the other (**Figure 10A**; white arrow heads). The giardial lesion alters the cytoskeleton of the colonic wall and the mode of intestinal peristalsis [3, 4]. The wall shows a concave contour and a "defect" during asymmetrical contraction (**Figure 10A**; top white arrow head). This is followed by relaxation and expansion into the preceding segment, in other words, by retropulsion (**Figure 10B**; white arrow) due to the defective intestinal motility [4].

In some patients, within the segment there is a dangling echogenic sheath, that falls short of the opposite wall, creating free-end septation with residual aperture (**Figure 10B**; double white small arrows). This sheath or septum is described as pseudo-haustration, since it lacked the oppositional arrangement of normal haustration [4]. Furthermore, the sheaths differ in shape, contour, and echogenicity from normal haustra. The residual aperture between the end of the sheath and colonic wall does not alter between contraction (**Figure 10A**; double white small arrows) and relaxation (**Figure 10B**; double white small arrows). This raises the possibility of partial obstruction of movement of intestinal contents by these pseudo-haustrations. The echogenicity of these pseudo-haustrations appeared similar to that of the echogenic submucosa, and showed anatomic continuity from that layer (**Figure 10B**; white small arrow head), until the sheath protrudes through

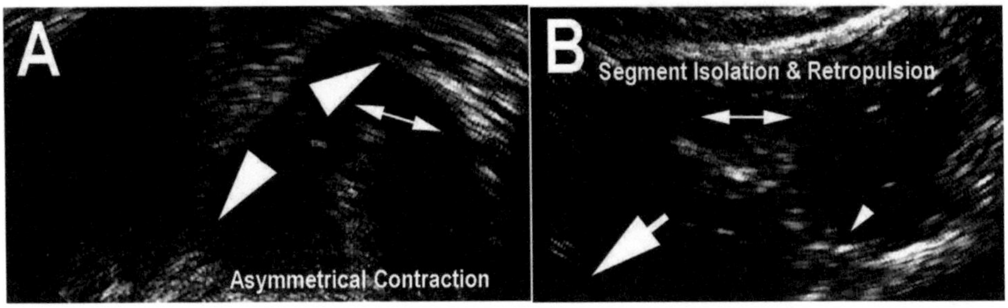

Figure 10.
Defective intestinal motility in giardiasis showing asymmetric contraction rings (A), followed by segment isolation and retropulsion (B).

the mucosal surface. This may suggest that these pseudo-haustrations derive from herniation of the submucosa through the mucosal surface (**Figure 10B**; white small arrow head) [4]. It has been suggested that a similar mechanism may result in invagination of the colonic wall after injury [6, 7].

4.3 Amebic lesions in the duodenum

In amebiasis, the duodenal wall thickness (5.4 ± 3 mm) is within normal limits [3, 4]. The wall echogenicity is usually not altered as seen in giardiasis. The folds of Kerkring have normal undulating contour. In contrast to giardiasis, in amebic lesion, HFF has increased echogenicity that moves slowly in bulk motion in helical fashion (**Figure 6C**).

4.4 Amebic lesions in the colon

Amebic lesions in the colon could be demonstrated using high-frequency B-mode ultrasound [8]. The wall thickness of the ascending colon (5.6 ± 3 mm) is marginally higher than in normal subjects but less than in patients with giardiasis [4]. There could be occasional collections demonstrated as well as delineated focal hyperechoic wall thickening lying on the mucosal surface (**Figure 11**, white arrow

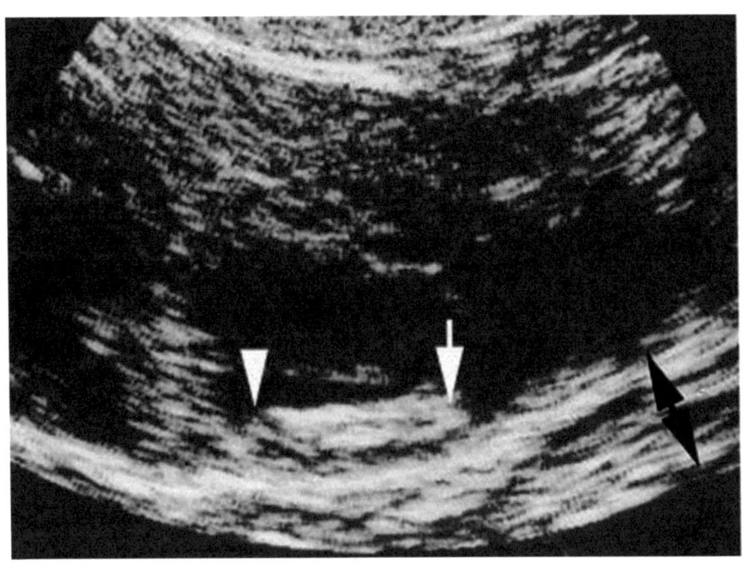

Figure 11.
Amebic abscess in the ascending colon with ameboma close to the haustra (between white arrow head and white arrow). The rest of the wall thickness remains within normal range (black double arrows).

heads). The focal thickening is associated with amebic granuloma (ameboma) and could be seen at the cecum, hepatic, and splenic flexures and sigmoid colon [4, 7]. It has been suggested that amebiasis may cause thickening of the submucosal layer due to hypervascularity of the bowel wall [8], but in contrast with generalized wall thickening observed in giardiasis, the changes in amebiasis are focal [4].

4.5 *Ancylostoma* in the duodenum

Ancylostoma duodenale and *Necator americanus* are nematode parasites that cause hookworm infection, and have a complex life cycle [9]. The mature *A. duodenale* female worms measure up to 15 mm (longer during blood meal), and the male worms up to 10 mm. *A. duodenale* could be demonstrated using high-frequency B-mode ultrasound as has been seen with gastroscopy [15]. The deep buccal cavity of the female worm could be clearly demonstrated with mouth parts and head visible in motion (**Figure 12A**, **B**, arrows). The visibility of the head and mouth parts could allow differentiation from other helminths, for example, the expected image of the male worm should show two spicules and the characteristic bursa. The mouth image of the female worm differs from the shallow buccal cavity of *Strongyloides stercoralis* [9]. The female worm become attached to the wall of the small intestine by sucking part of the mucosa into their mouth parts (**Figure 12C**), and abandoned sites (**Figure 12D**) continue to bleed [9]. The worm ingests blood from their host

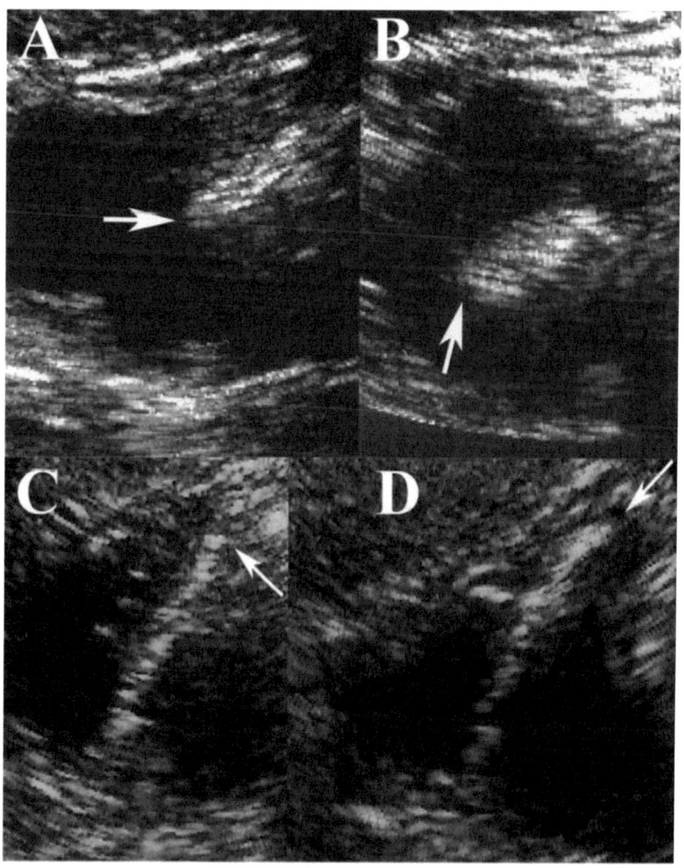

Figure 12.
Ancylostoma duodenale in the duodenum imaged in real-time with high-frequency B-mode ultrasound. The head and mouth parts move from one position (A) to another (B) to attach on the mucosal layer for blood meal (C, white arrow), and elongates and detaches thereafter (D, white arrow).

by the action of nematode anticoagulant protein c2 (NAPc2), a 85-amino acid protein with potent anticoagulant properties [16]. The process of ingestion of blood during a blood meal could be demonstrated using real-time high-frequency B-mode ultrasound. The worm is visualized in the proximal cephalid portion as a hyperechoic linear form (HLF) in active motion (**Figure 12A**, **B**, white arrow). The cephalid portion with two sharp pointed ends (buccal cavity) display jolting motility with jerking and leaping movements by spastic contractions and thickening (**Figure 12A**, **B**). The worm attaches to the mucosal surface at the duodenal near wall (**Figure 12C**). The worm could be observed attached to the mucosal layer (**Figure 12C**, white arrow) of the duodenum while ingesting blood. It could be seen elongating to about 20 mm in visible length, traversing the duodenal lumen. The caudal end lies in close proximity to the mucosal surface at the far wall. Under sonographic observation, the worm could be seen performing jolting motility, as it firmly attaches for a blood meal (**Figure 12C**, white arrow). It could be observed that as the worm elongates during a blood meal the entire visible length becomes hyperechoic. The proximal cephalid portion detaches from the mucosal surface (**Figure 12D**, white arrow) after the blood meal and the echogenicity of the worm changes with the upper one-third hyperechoic and the lower two-third hypoechoic. The latter is related to the movement of sucked blood through the gut of the worm. Stool analysis is used to reveal the eggs of *Ancylostoma duodenale* [9].

5. Common pitfalls of high-frequency ultrasound imaging of the intestine

1. Technical limitation of examination procedure due to abdominal tenderness, flatulence, or obesity.

2. Patient is unable to perform fasting due to health condition such as diabetes.

3. False negatives and false positives due to lack of proper technical access, condition of the patient, and similarity in motility patterns of the parasites.

4. Fluid filled bowel loops could alter the intestinal echoanatomy.

5. Constipation impairs bowel emptying and cause flatulence that technically impairs visualization due to fecal mass mimicking lesions in the intestine.

6. Large cystic lesions of the ovaries and fibromyoma may impair visualization of parts of the intestine.

7. Enlarged abdominal lymph nodes could also impair visualization of parts of the intestine.

8. Poor differentiations of colon cancer and lesions such as amebic abscess. However, the presence or absence of mesenteric lymph nodes and liver metastasis could aid differential diagnosis.

Author details

Philip C. Njemanze*, Josephine T. Njemanze, Clara C. Ofoegbu, Chinwendu C. Darlington, Esther Nneke, Ijeoma A. Onweni, Uchechi V. Ejiogu, Chinenye U. Mgbenu, Nneoma E. Ukeje, Anthonia C. Amadi and Doris C. Amaefule
Institute of Non-invasive Imaging for Parasitology, International Institutes of Advanced Research and Training, Chidicon Medical Center, Owerri, Imo State, Nigeria

*Address all correspondence to: philip.njemanze@chidicon.com

References

[1] World Health Organization Health Report. Conquering Suffering Enriching Humanity. Geneva: WHO; 1997. Available from: http://www.who.int/whr/1997/en/

[2] Delost MD. Introduction to Diagnostic Microbiology. St Louis: Mosby; 1997

[3] Njemanze PC, Anozie J, Chukwu C, Skelton A, Ogaraku AN. Ultrasound imaging characteristics of common protozoal and helminthic abdominal lesions. The American Journal of Tropical Medicine and Hygiene. 2001;**65**:205-206

[4] Njemanze PC, Njemanze J, Skelton A, Anoka A, Akagha O, Chukwu AA, et al. High-frequency ultrasound imaging of the duodenum and colon in patients with symptomatic giardiasis in comparison to amebiasis and healthy subjects. Journal of Gastroenterology and Hepatology. 2008;**23**:e37-e42. DOI: 1111/j.1440-1746.200705056.x

[5] Bowman WC, Rand MJ. Textbook of Pharmacology. 2nd ed. Vol. 1. Oxford: Blackwell Scientific Publications; 1980. pp. 25.24-25.30

[6] Gillespie IE, Thomson TJ. Gastroenterology: An Integrated Course. 3rd ed. Edinburgh: Churchill Livingstone; 1983. pp. 283-296

[7] Anderson WAD, Kissane JM. Pathology. 7th ed. Vol. 1. St Louis: CV Mosby; 1977. pp. 522-565

[8] Tsujimoto T, Kuriyama S, Yoshiji H, Fujimoto M, Kojima H, Yoshikawa M, et al. Ultrasonographic findings of amebic colitis. Journal of Gastroenterology. 2003;**38**:82-86

[9] Cheesbrough M. Medical Laboratory Manual for Tropical Countries. 2nd ed. Vol. 1. Oxford: ELBS with Tropical Health Technology/Butterworth-Heinemann Ltd.; 1992

[10] Choi D, Hong ST, Lim JH, et al. Sonographic findings of active *Clonorchis sinensis* infection. Journal of Clinical Ultrasound. 2004;**32**:17-23

[11] Mahmood T, Mansoor N, Quraishy S, Ilyas M, Hussain S. Ultrasonographic appearance of *Ascariasis lumbricoides* in the small bowel. Journal of Ultrasound in Medicine. 2001;**20**:269-274

[12] Wu S. Sonographic findings of *Ascariasis lumbricoides* in the gastrointestinal and biliary tracts. Ultrasound Quarterly. 2009;**25**:207-209. DOI: 10.1097/RUQ.0b013e3181c47a2d

[13] Galán-Puchades MT, Fuentes MV. The usefulness of ultrasound diagnosis specifically in taeniasis. Gut. 2008;**57**(515):524

[14] Areán VM, Koppisch E. Balantidiasis: A review and report of cases. The American Journal of Pathology. 1956;**32**:1089-1115

[15] Bamanikar S, Bamanikar A, Sawlani V, Pandit D. Gastroscopic diagnosis of ankylostoma duodenale infestation as a cause of iron-deficiency anemia. Medical Journal of Dr. D.Y. Patil Vidyapeeth University. 2014;**7**:631-633

[16] Lee AY, Vlasuk GP. Recombinant nematode anticoagulant protein c2 and other inhibitors targeting blood coagulation factor VIIa/tissue factor. Journal of Internal Medicine. 2003;**254**:313-321